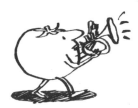

Samantha Heller not only gets it, she gets the details right. This is a funny, readable book spiced with great information on what you need to make healthy choices in nutrition, exercise, and lifestyle. We would all do well to follow her advice. Much more than just another diet book, *Get Smart* gives you the tools to make healthy choices.

**Edward K. Kasper, M.D.**
E. Cowles Professor in Cardiology
Director, Clinical Cardiology
Johns Hopkins Medical School

A book dedicated to keeping our minds fit and sharp with food—what a smart idea! Samantha Heller provides a wealth of information on how to nourish your brain with the right ingredients and offers fun, fresh meal ideas to get you off and running.

**Joy Bauer, M.S., R.D., C.D.N.**
*New York Times* bestselling author of *Your Inner Skinny*
Nutrition and diet expert for *The TODAY Show*

I am the Sneaky Chef, and I strongly recommend that you read this book! I am proud to have contributed recipes to it. As a mom, I am even more convinced by Samantha Heller's book that brain health is as much a factor of your lifestyle as the rest of your body's health. This book outlines a simple way to protect your brain, help prevent dementia, improve your mood, and enhance cognitive abilities at any age.

**Missy Chase Lapine**
Author of *The Sneaky Chef* books

Samantha Heller makes it easy to "get smart" and boost your brain power throughout your life cycle by following her user-friendly, realistic tips about what to put on your plate. This book will surely help you protect the organ that calls the shots about how you think, feel, act—and eat!

**Bonnie Taub-Dix, M.A., R.D., C.D.N.**
National Spokesperson for the American
Dietetic Association

Samantha Heller is a vibrant, passionate teacher. She is all about energy of the positive kind. Even better, she is an expert at where that energy comes from. That it can't be bottled, but that it can be developed. She knows the foods that contain this energy and she knows the combinations to the vault of good health. In *Get Smart*, she tells us her best secrets. We would be wise to listen.

**Marc Siegel, M.D.,** New York University
Medical director, Doctor Radio
Health columnist, *Los Angeles Times*
Fox News Medical Contributor

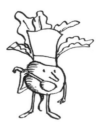

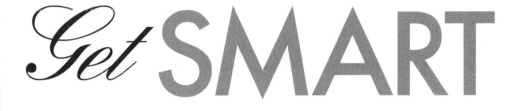

# Get SMART

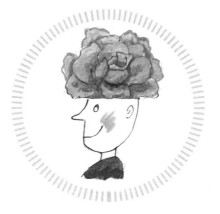

Samantha Heller's Nutrition Prescription
for Boosting Brain Power and Optimizing
Total Body Health

# Samantha Heller, M.S., R.D., C.D.N.

The Johns Hopkins University Press

BALTIMORE

**Notes to the reader:** Diet, exercise programs, and the use of medications are all matters that by their very nature vary from individual to individual. You should speak with your own doctor about your individual needs before beginning any diet or exercise program or taking any medications or other preparations. These precautionary notes are most important if you are already under medical care for an illness.

This book is not meant to substitute for medical care of people with cognitive difficulties, and treatment should not be based solely on its contents. Treatment for medical illness must be developed in a dialogue between the individual and his or her physician.

The Johns Hopkins University Press
2715 North Charles Street
Baltimore, Maryland 21218-4363
www.press.jhu.edu

**Recipes:** On pages 198–203, from *The Most Decadent Diet Ever!* by Devin Alexander. Copyright © 2008 by Devin Alexander. Reprinted with permission from Broadway Books, a Division of Random House, Inc., New York. On pages 193, 195–96, and 203–4, reprinted by permission of Barbara Smith. On pages 180–81 and 186–87, from *The Sneaky Chef: Simple Strategies for Hiding Healthy Foods in Kids' Favorite Meals*, by Missy Chase Lapine, copyright © 2007 by Running Press Book Publisher. On pages 181–82 and 205–7, reprinted by permission of Rosa J. Donohue, M.S., R.D., C.D.N., Nutrition Consultant. On pages 197–98, reprinted by permission of Frances Largeman-Roth, R.D. Recipes on pages 183–85, 188–93, 194–95, 204–5, and 207–9, reprinted by permission of Amie G. Hall, CHHC, AADP.

Illustrations by Joe Weissmann.

**Library of Congress Cataloging-in-Publication Data**

Heller, Samantha.
   Get smart : Samantha Heller's nutrition prescription for boosting brain power and achieving total body health / Samantha Heller.
      p. cm.
   Includes bibliographical references and index.
ISBN-13: 978-0-8018-9375-9 (hardcover : alk. paper)
ISBN-10: 0-8018-9375-5 (hardcover : alk. paper)
ISBN-13: 978-0-8018-9376-6 (pbk. : alk. paper)
ISBN-10: 0-8018-9376-3 (pbk. : alk. paper)
   1. Brain. 2. Nutrition. 3. Brain chemistry. 4. Mental health—Nutritional aspects. I. Title.
QP376.H317 2009
612.8'2—dc22          2009007055

A catalog record for this book is available from the British Library.

*Special discounts are available for bulk purchases of this book. For more information, please contact Special Sales at 410-516-6936 or specialsales@press.jhu.edu.*

The Johns Hopkins University Press uses environmentally friendly book materials, including recycled text paper that is composed of at least 30 percent post-consumer waste, whenever possible. All of our book papers are acid-free, and our jackets and covers are printed on paper with recycled content.

*To my mother, Terry Strong Heller, for her grace, intelligence, dignity, and humor*

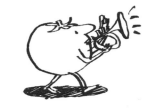

# Contents

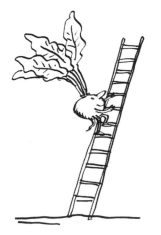

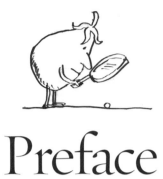

# Preface

FRED CAME INTO MY office for his appointment and said, "Look, I need to lose weight. Just give me a diet."

"No, Fred, I do not hand out diets."

He looked at me and asked, carefully, "Then what do you do?"

"Fred," I said, "I don't believe in dieting. The word *diet* instills fear and loathing in people. It means temporary, hungry, and deprived. My goal is to first, teach you what healthy eating is, and second, give you the tools you need to make healthy choices on a daily basis. Together you and I will create meal plans based on foods you like and have available at work and at home."

Fred was not thrilled with that approach. He wanted something simple, in print, that he could follow for a week or two. A standard 1,200 or 1,500 calorie per day diet does not work, because everyone has different needs. Plus, a cookie-cutter diet does not take into account your life, where you work, food allergies, social situations, traveling, and such. Healthy lifestyle choices need to fit in with your food preferences, budget, and work and home schedule. These choices have to work for you so you can keep them the rest of your life.

Your assignment (should you choose to accept it) is to take the information in this book and mold it to fit your world. Will changing your current eating habits and lifestyle take some discipline and thought?

Definitely. Will there be times when it seems hard to stick to a healthy-brain eating plan? Yes. But that's OK. Just keep referring to this book for support and advice. You may consider seeing a registered dietitian if you really get stuck. Since you are reading this book in the first place, you are motivated to make some changes for a healthier brain.

Why not start right now?

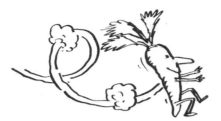

# Acknowledgments

MY ETERNAL THANKS TO my patients, students, colleagues, family, and friends who share their knowledge, experiences, and stories with me and from whom I continue to learn so much. My thanks to Jacqueline Wehmueller, executive editor at the Johns Hopkins University Press, who saw promise in the book, offered thoughtful advice and expertise, and gave a first-time author a chance. To all the people at the Johns Hopkins University Press who had a hand in helping create the final book, I offer my thanks and appreciation for their expertise. I'd like to thank journalist and friend Colette Bouchez, who has been pushing me to write a book for a long time and who has given her continual support peppered with a great deal of irreverent humor.

A huge thank-you to the chefs who donated their delicious recipes to this book. Without exception or hesitation, each chef offered to share her recipes with great generosity and enthusiasm. Thank you to Devin Alexander, Missy Chase Lapine, Amie Guyette Hall, Rosa J. Donohue, Frances Largeman-Roth, and B. Smith.

## A Personal Note

MY MOM HAS DEMENTIA. She does not have Alzheimer's disease. Alzheimer's is just one of several forms of dementia. At this writing she is 90 years old. I visit her in the nursing home every day. Her dementia is confusing for me. Some days she can be lucid, insightful, even funny. Very Mom-like. Other days she is very confused, depressed, and muddled. She knows where she is and does not understand why she cannot come live with me. Mom says the people who live on her unit are "crazy." She's right, of course; she is on a dementia unit. Mom follows me to the door when I leave. When it closes, she puts her hand up to the glass. I put mine up to hers and we say goodbye.

It took me a long time to fully accept her diagnosis of dementia. It is not that I was in denial (I don't think). I thought her confusion was related to poor vision and hearing. In retrospect I realize that her decline began many years ago. The signs were so subtle.

Am I at risk? I do not know. Doctors don't know. Mom smoked for many years but did not eat badly. She did not eat particularly well, either. She exercised on and off. I think it was the smoking that contributed to her dementia and high blood pressure. Of course high blood pressure also affects brain function. By following my own advice, the Get Smart Nutrition Prescription for Boosting Brain Power and Optimizing Total Body Health, I am lowering the risk of developing dementia as well as the many chronic diseases that contribute to the development of cognitive decline and dementia. Maintaining a healthy lifestyle also helps mood, energy, and coping skills. You feel better, think better, and have more fun.

# Get SMART

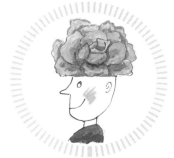

# Introduction

HAVE YOU EVER LOOKED up while driving and wondered where you were and how you got there? Walked into a room and forgot why? What about when you left the potted begonia you just bought on the top of the car and drove off? You worry that perhaps these are signs of early dementia but then reassure yourself that it is just normal wear and tear due to stress and fatigue. You are not the only one experiencing memory glitches, foggy thoughts, and confused moments. As the population ages, these experiences and the worries that accompany them are becoming more common. In this regard, here are some facts to consider:

- There are 78.2 million baby boomers in the United States.
- Approximately 500,000 people under the age of 65 have been diagnosed with early-onset Alzheimer's or other dementias.
- People of all ages complain about memory loss, inability to focus, mood swings, and forgetfulness.
- Brain health is directly related to nutrition and lifestyle.
- A healthy lifestyle can reduce the risk of, delay, and maybe even prevent chronic diseases like heart disease, diabetes, cancer, stroke, and obesity, all of which have a profound impact on brain health.
- A healthy lifestyle can improve memory, mental clarity, energy, and mood.

The baby boomer generation is dealing with aging parents and seeing firsthand how devastating mental and cognitive decline is for everyone involved. Premenopausal women complain about memory loss and poor focus. Mothers joke that having children kills brain cells, but they aren't really kidding. They are physically sleep deprived and mentally overstretched. Behavioral problems, which research suggests are strongly affected by diet, are on the increase in kids, teens, young adults, and politicians. (Oh come on. All politicians behave badly.) The boomers in particular, but also younger professionals and parents, are desperate to learn how to boost their brain power, make smarter babies, get teens to do better in school, and excel in their careers. People are concerned with what might happen to their brain as they age. In its 2008 *Pfizer Australia Health Report*, the drug company Pfizer reported its finding that almost three-quarters (74%) of all Australians would take a test (if it was available) to find out—*before* they started experiencing signs or symptoms—whether they are going to develop dementia. It is a safe bet to say that most people would really like to know what they need to do to get a healthy brain. *Get Smart* offers in-depth information and realistic brain-health advice that can be incorporated into daily life.

The Alzheimer's Association predicts that with the nation's 78 million baby boomers beginning to turn 60 in 2006, by midcentury someone will develop Alzheimer's every 33 seconds. Worldwide, there is a new case of dementia every seven seconds. It is unnerving to discover that the rate of dementia is expected to double between 2001 and 2040 in developed nations and it is forecast to increase by more than 300 percent in India and China. Clearly, there is a desperate need for us to learn how to reduce the risk of developing Alzheimer's and other forms of dementia and improve our overall health. Aside from diagnosable brain problems, many people are experiencing a general mental malaise. Poor focus, poor memory, and forgetfulness are common among people of all ages. Nutrition and lifestyle throughout the life cycle play critical roles in reaching and maintaining brain health. *Get Smart* details—in practical, easy-to-understand language—what can be done to reduce the risk of cognitive decline and dementia and what you can do to boost memory, mental clarity, and overall mood.

*Get Smart* is not just about dodging dementia by having a healthy brain. It is also about having a healthy body. You cannot have one without the other. With obesity rates soaring, heart disease the number one killer in the United States, and diabetes hitting epidemic levels, it is no wonder that approximately 500,000 people under age 65 have been diagnosed with some type of dementia. Diabetes, heart disease, and obesity are significant factors in the development of cognitive problems. Choosing a lifestyle that reduces the risks of these diseases translates to a healthier brain. The human brain is capable of performing 20 million billion calculations per second, but if it is not well nourished or the body is diseased, the brain is at higher risk for cognitive impairment or dementia. A healthy lifestyle may be able to delay, reduce, or prevent the risk of developing dementia and improve mood, relieve depression and anxiety, and enhance cognitive capabilities.

It is never too early to start good brain nutrition. Everyone wants healthy children, but few parents are aware that poor nutrition in children as young as 3 years of age can lead to later antisocial and aggressive behavior. *Get Smart* offers healthy eating tips for the whole family.

It is never too late to start good brain nutrition, either. Studies show that those who adopt a healthy lifestyle in middle age experience "prompt" benefits in their health. In healthy elderly people, improving cognitive performance can be as simple as eating a potato.

This book explains what you need to do to improve brain health, heart health, psychological well-being, and energy levels—and why. As an educator I feel it is very important to understand *why* certain recommendations are made. If you understand *why* a food or behavior is good or bad for you, it is easier to make changes. (If you do not care about the *why*, you can skip the explanations and just read the bulleted points and the summaries in each chapter.)

The program is flexible, so you can adapt it to fit your budgetary needs and cultural and food preferences. If you can't afford Atlantic salmon, canned will do just as well. If you were raised on white rice and beans, switch over to brown rice and use canola oil instead of animal fat in the refried beans. If your neighborhood bodega does not have fresh vegetables, frozen will do nicely. If you absolutely have to have pizza for lunch, get a slice (or two) with all vegetables, low-fat or no cheese (it's delicious, try it).

While most people think they know what a healthy lifestyle is and what foods are healthy, decisions about food and health are usually far more complex than people realize. José, a small wiry man in his forties, had come to see me for nutrition counseling. He had heart disease. José told me he had spent several years cooking heart-healthy meals for his wife, who had type 2 diabetes.

"But I ate differently myself," he noted.

"Tell me what you have been eating," I asked.

"You won't like it," he cautioned.

"Try me."

"I . . ." He searched for the word. "You know butter?"

"Yes," I responded encouragingly. "You use butter."

"No, you do not understand. I have butter with white bread."

"Ok, you put butter on bread. I understand that."

"No," he repeated. "I take a whole stick of butter, wrap a piece of bread around it, and eat it."

At that point I was speechless.

This is not a diet book. This book is designed to give you the tools you need to make healthy choices that will improve brain and total body health and fitness. The scientific research studies on which the recommendations are based were done on humans, not on animals or cells in test tubes. The reason is that research done on animals or in test tubes cannot be extrapolated to humans, so I do not feel it is valid to use these types of research as the basis for diet or lifestyle recommendations. In addition, I am against animal testing. It is unnecessary and cruel.

Since this is not a diet book, I have not laid out specific weekly meal plans. There are many meal and snack suggestions, shopping lists, tips, and delicious recipes for you to use to create your own nutrition prescription. The more personalized you make your plan, the easier it will be to make choices to be healthy every day.

## *Get Smart*'s Basic Nutrition Prescription for Boosting Brain Power and Optimizing Total Body Health

### The Yes's

- Eat a lot of vegetables every single day. Raw, sautéed, nuked, steamed. Any way you like them, except deep fried. Aim for 9–11 servings each day. One serving of vegetables is ½ cup cooked or 1 cup raw. Most people don't actually count their servings of vegetables, so just be sure to have vegetables at lunch and dinner daily, and if you can throw some in at breakfast and with snacks, that's good too.
- Eat 2 to 3 fruits a day. One serving of fruit is 1 piece of fruit, 1 cup of berries, ½ grapefruit.
- Choose whole grains like whole-wheat pasta, brown and wild rices, whole-grain cereals. Whole grains are an excellent source of energy and healthy nutrients. Watch your portion sizes, though. The USDA recommends about 5–6 servings a day. One serving is about 1 ounce, which = 1 slice of bread, ½ cup of cooked pasta, 1 cup of cereal, or 1 6″ tortilla. The reality is that no one eats only ½ cup of pasta. One cup is more reasonable. Fill it out with a ton of vegetables, and you have a nice healthy meal. Just be aware of how many servings of grains you have in a day. They add up quickly.
- Use healthy oils like olive, canola, peanut, sesame, and walnut oils daily.
- Eat only lean, healthy sources of protein like low-fat or nonfat dairy, soy, nuts, egg whites, and beans.
- If you choose to eat animal foods, select white-meat skinless poultry or fish. Two 3- to 4-ounce portions a day is the general recommendation.
- Nibble on some dark chocolate for fun.
- Exercise every day. Dance, hop, jump, anything. At least 30 minutes. But every bit of exercise, even a 10-minute walk, is good.
- Challenge your brain regularly with new skills, tasks, games, and knowledge.
- Go organic and support local farmers whenever you can.

- Be social. Talk to friends. Visit neighbors. Join a book club. Volunteer at your local school to read to kids. Socializing stimulates the brain and may delay cognitive decline. Besides, it's fun. Studies indicate that a socially integrated lifestyle may protect against dementia and Alzheimer's disease.

## The No's

- Stay away from saturated fat, red meat, and processed meats.
- Never eat trans fats or hydrogenated oils (they are the same thing).
- Avoid white flour, white rice and pasta, cookies, cakes, sweets, pastries.
- Dump the soda and sweetened drinks such as iced teas and fruit drinks.
- Do not overeat.
- Steer clear of fast food and junk food.
- Limit alcohol.
- Do not isolate yourself.
- Quit smoking. You can do it. It is your choice. There are aids to help you quit smoking such as patches, gums, and medications. Try a smoking cessation or support group.

## Art Isn't Easy

The art of personalizing your nutrition prescription and incorporating healthy changes into your life will be challenging at first. TV ads, food courts at the mall, the bakery at the grocery store (notice how good it smells right when you walk in the door—that is not an accident), and family-style cheap meals conspire to sabotage someone who is trying to make choices for health every day. You may also find that friends and family do not seem supportive of the changes you are trying to make. Don't take it personally. Change can be difficult for everyone. This is not unusual. Start by bringing in one or two healthy choices at each meal, slowly decreasing the unhealthy foods like butter, cheese, and red meat. Of course, once or twice a month it's OK to indulge in some of the foods you miss.

Sharpening your brain will not happen with just one change, like skipping a lunchtime soda. It takes a whole lifestyle makeover to create the physical environment your brain and body need to be focused, clear, quick, and healthy. You can jump in with both feet using the Two-Week Kick Start Plan, or you can start one step at a time. You can choose how you want to start by reading through the chapters and seeing which healthy step you feel like taking today. Perhaps you will have a whole-grain cereal for breakfast instead of a cheese Danish. Or healthy no-cheese vegetable pizza for lunch instead of a roast beef sandwich. Maggie, a 24-year-old patient, is working on Wall Street, so her days are crazy. She takes clients out to eat often, works 12 hours a day, and is about to get married. She wants to lose weight before her wedding. She and I are trying to create a healthy eating plan that she can manage with this stressful schedule. I suggested the healthy pizza as one option for her.

"Uh yeah," she agreed, not wanting to offend me. "I, uh, yeah. I guess I could try that."

"It's really good," I assured her.

She was clearly unconvinced. When I saw her a week later, though, she told me, "I went to California Pizza Kitchen and got an all-vegetable, no-cheese pizza. It was delicious! I never would have thought to do that before!"

Take time to break out of old habits and patterns. A healthy brain needs change and stimulation. Just by making the changes suggested in this book you will be offering your brain a challenge. You will be looking at food in new ways, trying new foods, managing eating out and social occasions from a healthy-brain point of view, and preparing meals differently. Your brain and your body will thank you. When you begin the Get Smart lifestyle, you could start feeling better in as little as two weeks. In one study patients were given a brain-healthy diet, relaxation exercises, cardiovascular conditioning, and mental exercises like brain teasers. After only 14 days these patients showed significant improvements in cognitive function and brain metabolism.

There is no time like the present to Get Smart with your own nutrition prescription for boosting brain power and optimizing total body health.

# What Are Alzheimer's Disease and Dementia?

*The Alzheimer's Association describes Alzheimer's disease as a progressive brain disorder that gradually destroys a person's memory and ability to learn, reason, make judgments, communicate, and carry out daily activities.*

*Alzheimer's disease is a type of dementia. Not all people suffering from cognitive decline or dementia develop Alzheimer's. Early dementia may be characterized by forgetfulness, difficulty with familiar tasks, trouble finding words, behavioral or personality changes, or impaired judgment.*

*The Canadian Study of Health and Aging reports that increasing age, fewer years of education, and the apolipoprotein E$\varepsilon$4 allele (a gene) were significantly associated with increased risk of Alzheimer's disease. Use of nonsteroidal anti-inflammatory drugs, wine consumption, coffee consumption, and regular physical activity were associated with a reduced risk of Alzheimer's disease. Research suggests that greater education is associated with a lower risk of dementia, but scientists are not sure why. They hypothesize that more highly educated persons may have a greater cognitive reserve that can postpone the clinical manifestation of dementia. Unhealthy lifestyles may independently contribute to the depletion of this reserve or directly influence the underlying pathologic processes.*

*Consult a doctor when you have concerns about memory loss, thinking skills, and behavior changes in yourself or a loved one. (See also www.alz.org/alzheimers_disease_what_is_alzheimers.asp)*

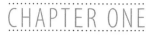

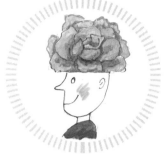

## CHAPTER ONE

# The Fat Head

————— KEY POINTS —————

⇨ Two-thirds of the brain is made up of fat.

⇨ There are 100 billion neurons.

⇨ The protective covering of nerve cells called myelin is 70 percent fat.

⇨ The brain uses dietary fatty acids by incorporating them into cell membranes.

⇨ You need to eat certain fats for a healthy brain.

⇨ Bad fats can get incorporated into the brain and central nervous system and impair function.

⇨ Trans and saturated fats may increase the risk of cognitive decline and dementia.

⇨ Good fats that come from plants and seafood are critical for a healthy brain.

———— NUTRITION PRESCRIPTION ————
*for* FATS

⇨ **Include healthy fats in your diet daily. These include plant oils such as olive, canola, peanut, and sesame oils and foods such as avocados and nuts.**

⇨ **Eat only low-fat or nonfat dairy foods like nonfat milk, cheese, and cottage cheese.**

⇨ **Avoid red and processed meats, saturated and trans fats.**

⇨ **Be sure to eat foods high in omega-3 fats: soy, walnuts, ground flaxseeds, fish.**

**Brain Facts:** The human brain weighs between 1,300 and 1,400 grams. A stegosaurus dinosaur weighed approximately 1,600 kilograms but had a brain that weighed only about 70 grams.

YOU ARE AT DINNER with a friend, and a woman in the Pilates class that you have been taking for eight months comes up to say hello. Just as you are about to introduce her to your friend, you realize you cannot remember her name. Mortified, you skip the introductions and launch into a conversation about the Pilates instructor's recent Botox debacle. After you say your good-byes and she leaves, you apologize to your dining companion for not introducing her. Several hours later while flossing your teeth, you suddenly exclaim, "Margo! Her name is Margo!"

The human body is run primarily by two systems: the endocrine system and the nervous system. The endocrine system uses hormones to do its job, which is mostly to regulate the body's metabolic functions. The nervous system involves the brain and spinal cord and more than 100 billion neurons. The nervous system helps control all the body's systems, organs, sensations, thoughts, memory, and appetite; it directs communications and performs a zillion other tasks. We do not generally associate the brain or neurons with fats (also known as lipids or fatty acids), yet the nervous system has the second-highest tissue concentration of fats in the body (the highest concentration is in adipose tissue, or fat cells). Many neurons are sheathed in a substance called myelin, which is about 70 percent fat and helps with signal conduction. Neurons can send signals to thousands of other cells at 200 miles per hour. The kind of fats you eat will make a difference in how well and how fast your neurons communicate. Good fats can give you NASCAR neurons, and bad fats will give you junky jalopies. There are several different kinds of lipids that are required components in both the structure and function of the brain.

The availability of fats to the brain depends on what you eat every day. These fats will affect how well the brain functions.

It is only a slight stretch to say that if you'd eaten oatmeal for breakfast instead of a cheese Danish, you may have remembered Margo's name more easily. Realistically, if you have been eating breakfast pastries, sausage and egg sandwiches, and sugar-coated cereals for years, or skipping breakfast altogether, chances are the neurons in your brain are not communicating effectively. The reason is that more than two-thirds of the brain is made up of fat, and the *type* of fat you eat has a direct effect on how well the brain functions over time.

One cheese Danish won't Taser every thought in your head, but years of eating bad fats and refined foods can significantly alter brain function.

One day at the gym, years ago (before I became a nutritionist), my friend Maria, who read a lot of magazines, told me that she had read that eating fat was a very bad thing and we should all go fat free. That sounded reasonable to me because trying to lose fat is what drove me to the gym in the first place. Apparently, the notion of "fat free" made sense to a lot of people, since it spawned thousands of "fat free" diet books and cookbooks. All these years later I still encounter resistance, even fear, when I try to encourage people to add healthy fats to their diets. The truth is, we need fat to have a healthy body and brain. The problem is we have been eating a lot of bad fats that are not good for the brain and too much fat altogether.

It is easy to get confused when discussing fats—partly because there are many kinds of fats that have different functions and effects in the body and partly because nutrition is all about chemistry, which most of us skipped out of in high school. Simply put, there are good fats and bad fats and fats we cannot live without called essential fatty acids. To get the essential fatty acids into our bodies we must eat them. Other fats, like cholesterol, are made in the body. And some fats are made up of other nutrients. Eventually fats get into the bloodstream, circulate throughout the body, and become incorporated into brain and nervous tissues, arteries, cells, and organs. This chapter will tell you everything you need to know about fats and why you need to know—why bad fats are bad and good fats are good and what to eat to optimize your brain power.

---

There are good fats and bad fats. They all have direct effects in the body. Eating good fats from foods like nuts and avocados and using olive oil will help your brain rock and roll. Eating bad fats like butter, red meat, and cheese regularly can reduce your brain power to a polka, in slow motion, in a snowstorm.

---

## Good Fat, Bad Fat

Good, work-healthy fats:

- help absorb vitamins A, D, E, and K;
- are critical for a healthy brain and central nervous system;
- boost immune function;
- keep skin healthy;
- help manage the healing process;
- pad and protect our bodies;
- taste really good; and
- provide energy.

"You're trying to kill us!" one woman exclaimed when I suggested that she and her husband, who had had a heart attack, try hummus as a snack. Hummus is a delicious combination of pureed chickpeas, tahini (sesame paste), garlic, olive oil, lemon juice, and other flavors and makes a great dip for vegetables. "Hummus has *fat* in it," she said accusingly. The whole nutrition class erupted in a heated debate over whether I was trying to kill them all. It took the better part of an hour to calm the woman down. It is not surprising that she was confused about fat, as are most people. The U.S. Department of Agriculture, American Heart Association, American Cancer Society, American Diabetes Association, and many other organizations all recommend that we reduce our intake of saturated fats, trans fats, and cholesterol. The problem is most of us have no idea what saturated fats, trans fats, and cholesterol are, what they do, or in what foods they are found, so we just assume that all fats are deadly. For a healthy, well-functioning brain and cardiovascular system we need to figure out the difference between good and bad fats. We want to eat the good ones and avoid the bad ones. I don't know whether the fat-phobic woman was ever convinced that some fats are not only good for you but critical for survival, but I did my best.

Before we go into good and bad fats, you need to know a little bit about inflammation, how it affects your brain and body, and the roles different fats play in the process of inflammation.

You know what inflammation feels like. A burned hand, a blistered heel from new shoes (Jimmy Choo's or Payless), a sore throat, or aching joints are all the result of inflammation. Inflammation is the body's natural immune response to injury, infection, or trauma. Acute inflammation is characterized by redness, swelling, heat, and pain. Inflammation helps heal by sending white and red blood cells and special chemicals to the problem area to fight infectious agents, repair damaged tissues, eliminate toxins, signal the body to clot blood, and knit tissues back together. Fats play a central role in the process of inflammation and healing. The kind of fat you eat can hasten these processes or inhibit them.

Calling someone a "hothead" may not be far from the truth. Scientists now believe that chronic inflammation affects brain health. Chronic inflammation means that something in the body, like arteries, neurons, or tissues, is being constantly irritated. This continual irritation causes the inflammation process to go haywire. The result is a buildup of sludge, plaque, and other goo that interferes with the function of arteries and neurons and with circulation and other physiological processes. We know that inflammation is the cornerstone of many chronic diseases such as heart disease, diabetes, arthritis, and cancer. Now, emerging research is telling us that inflammation damages not only our joints, blood vessels, and organs but the brain and nervous system too. What causes chronic inflammation? What we eat, stress levels, environment, and lifestyle can all increase *or* decrease systemic inflammation.

Fats are directly involved in the process of inflammation. Inflammation contributes to many chronic diseases. The type of fats and foods you eat affects how your body handles inflammation. Good fats reduce inflammation. Bad fats like saturated and trans increase it. Inflammation is a key suspect in the development of Alzheimer's disease and other forms of dementia. Whether you are 1 or 100 years old, if you don't want your brain to become a junk pile of inflammatory sludge, it is important to nourish it with the right fats.

## Oxidative Dancing

Buff men. Scantily clad women. Sequined gowns and stilettos cha-cha-ing all over the place. The TV phenomenon *Dancing with the Stars* has ignited a whole new interest in partnered dance. Whether you are jitterbugging or doing the mambo, it's fun and phenomenal exercise. What would happen, though, if all the partners disappeared the day of the big competition? You'd see single dancers desperately looking for another partner. They'd start grabbing anyone who came along and try to dance with him or her. It could get ugly. Imagine Mario Lopez flipping former first lady Laura Bush over his shoulders and between his legs. Basically, that is what oxidative stress is. Oxygen molecules that have an unpaired electron (the single dancer) are called oxidants, or free radicals. They desperately need to latch on to another molecule that has an available electron (the partner). In the brain and body the formation

*The* 2008 Dancing with the Stars *season featured Oscar award–winning actress Cloris Leachman as a contestant. She was 82 at the start of the show. Ms. Leachman's youthful energy can most likely be attributed to a healthy vegetarian diet and a lifetime of regular physical activity. (If you do not know who Cloris Leachman is, watch the original film of* Young Frankenstein. *She plays Frau Blucher.)*

of oxidants, or free radicals, is a normal part of daily life. But when too many oxidants (single dancers) are produced, they start latching on to anything they can, such as cells, DNA, protein, and fats. That is when damage and inflammation occur. Along come the antioxidants to save the day. They pair up with the oxidants and waltz off into the sunset. Antioxidants like vitamins C and E, selenium, and beta carotene are happy to join the dance and stop the insanity.

Excess oxidants are formed as a result of poor diet, illness, pollution, smoking, aging, and low levels of antioxidants. Scientists believe that oxidative damage is a significant contributor to brain aging and cognitive decline. *Get Smart* focuses on foods that decrease oxidative damage, such as healthy fats, fruits, and vegetables. These foods contain antioxidants that help reduce oxidative damage and protect and repair damaged cells.

Oxidative damage can be minimized with a healthy diet and lifestyle.

☞ Inflammation is the cornerstone of many diseases.

☞ Eating foods that reduce internal inflammation may lower the risk of cognitive decline and chronic diseases such as heart disease, arthritis, diabetes, and cancer.

☞ Cardiovascular disease and diabetes affect cognitive function.

☞  Oxidative stress contributes to aging brains and bodies, inflammation, and disease.

☞  Eating foods high in antioxidants helps reduce damage caused by oxidative stress.

## Good Fats

There are lots of things to know about good fats.

- Good fats are unsaturated and essential for a healthy brain and body.
- You have to eat essential fatty acids (EFA) for them to be used by the body.
- Unsaturated fats (mono- and polyunsaturated) help improve brain function, reduce the risk of diseases, and have anti-inflammatory properties.
- The growth and development of the fetus and placenta are dependent on the mother eating enough essential fatty acids.
- Fish, soy, tofu, walnuts, flaxseed oil, and seaweed are good food sources of omega-3 fatty acids.
- Vegetables, nuts, seeds, and whole grains have healthy fats.
- Eating good fats may ultimately help you remember your friend's name.

Hallelujah, fat is good! Pull out the organic extra virgin olive, expeller-pressed canola, walnut, flaxseed, sesame, and peanut oils and have a fat fest. While it is true that fat has more calories (9 calories per gram) than protein or carbohydrates (4 calories per gram each), it is also true that there are certain fats called essential fatty acids that we cannot live without. The only way to get these essential fatty acids into our bodies is to eat them. The brain is dependent on the fats you eat to keep it healthy. A diet low in these essential fats diminishes the concentrations in the brain and causes neurochemical and behavioral changes. The "no fat" fad diets of the past are not only passé; they are downright unhealthy. Fats help us absorb vitamins, work in the immune and central nervous systems, keep cells healthy, and are important contributors to the formation of vitamin D and hormones. Not eating enough good fat can put a serious dent in the body's ability to function properly.

Studies are telling us that replacing saturated fat, a bad fat, with healthy unsaturated fats can reduce our risk of chronic diseases and help manage weight. Replacing butter with olive oil, frozen yogurt with fat-free frozen yogurt, and using a balsamic vinaigrette instead of blue cheese dressing are steps in the right direction. And let's face it, fat makes food taste good. Adding healthy fats to your diet is a win-win situation.

Good fats are unsaturated, liquid at room temperature, and generally come from plants. These healthy fats include olive, canola, walnut, peanut, sesame, flaxseed, and avocado oils. But not all fats that come from plants are healthy—coconut, palm, and palm kernel oils are saturated, solid at room temperature, and just as bad for you as butter and lard. Cocoa butter, the foundation for chocolate, is a saturated fat too, but it does not seem to have the unhealthy effects of its saturated sisters (if you think for a moment . . . this means that you can eat dark chocolate occasionally guilt free).

---

Healthy fats, like olive, canola, walnut, sesame, and soy oils, are unsaturated and come from plants. They are found in foods like fish, nuts, avocados, seeds (sunflower, pumpkin), tofu, and ground flax-seeds. Healthy fats reduce inflammation, boost our immune system, make our arteries and brain cells happy. And our taste buds too.

---

**Foods with Good Fats**
    Fish
    Avocado
    Nuts (all of them, unsalted)
    Seeds
    Flaxseeds (ground)
    Flaxseed oil
    Soy, tofu

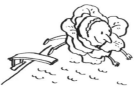

## Sisters, Cousins, and Aunts

**Chemical Facts about Fats:** Saturated fats have no double bonds, are totally saturated with hydrogens, and are solid at room temperature. Unsaturated fats have one or more double bonds. They have room for the double bonds because they have fewer hydrogens on them. Unsaturated fats are liquid at room temperature.

Within the unsaturated fat family there are many relatives. In the movie *My Big Fat Greek Wedding* Toula is on a date with her WASPy new beau, Ian. "How many cousins do you have?" she asks. "Two," he replies. She just looks at him. "I have 27 first cousins. Just 27 first cousins alone!" You could say that the unsaturated fat family is like Toula's family, with a ton of first, second, and third cousins. There is a large family of cousins in the world of fats, and it can be confusing to figure out who's who in the fat family. You have heard of mono- and polyunsaturated fats. You really do not need to worry about the difference because you need both types of fats to be healthy. The key here is the word *UNsaturated*. This means they are good for you. Within each of the mono- and polyunsaturated fat groups there are subgroups, the cousins.

On the polyunsaturated side of the family there are two omega-3 fatty acids known as DHA (docosahexaenoic acid) and EPA (eicosentaenoic acid). These are the family favorites and are found in fish, walnuts, soy, canola oil, flaxseed oil, and greens like purslane. There are also the omega-6 and omega-9 fatty acids that are needed for a healthy body. The 6s and 9s are found in foods such as sunflower and sesame oils, macadamia nuts, and pecans. All of these unsaturated fats play important roles throughout life, from brain development in fetuses to keeping aging brains functioning at their best. Think of the omegas as third, sixth, and ninth cousins in a family.

You have heard of the health benefits of the Mediterranean diet. This diet is characterized by monounsaturated oils found in avocado and olive oil. Monounsaturated oils, the sisters to polyunsaturated oils, are also in foods like olive and peanut oils.

Now that you know how good unsaturated fats are for you, you can finally give up your fear of fat. It can be confusing, but just think "plant fat good, animal fat bad." Roger, a patient of mine, was very attached to the idea that all fat was bad. When I suggested he have a peanut butter and jelly sandwich for lunch instead of his usual burger and fries, he looked at me like I was a quack. "But peanut butter has fat in it!" "Yes it does. But it is a good fat," I entreated. He remained skeptical. "You can lead a horse to water . . ."

Unsaturated fats are good and come from plants. Polyunsaturated cousins omega-3, -6, and -9 and the monounsaturated fats are necessary for good health. They are found in many foods including wheat germ (great in yogurt), halibut, winter squash, and pistachios.

Good Stuff about eating unsaturated fats:

- Unsaturated fats appear to be protective against Alzheimer's and cognitive decline.
- Unsaturated fats may have a protective effect against Parkinson's disease.
- Higher intake of unsaturated fats is associated with improved performance in kids.
- The anti-inflammatory activity of HDL cholesterol (the good cholesterol) improves after consumption of unsaturated fat.
- Unsaturated fats lower bad cholesterol (LDL) and raise good cholesterol (HDL).
- Eating unsaturated fats instead of saturated fats (animal fat) lowers the risk of cardiovascular disease and protects the heart.
- Monounsaturated oils have been found to be protective against age-related cognitive decline and are heart healthy.

## The Balance of 3s and 6s

I was at Sears in the mall with my friend Shelia trying to decide between a less expensive vacuum cleaner and one that had more features for more money when behind me I heard someone call out Shelia's name. This woman came bounding up and gushed, "Oh my gosh! I have not seen you in *soooo* long. You look amazing!" She turned to her husband and said, "You remember Shelia? She came to our Christmas party a few years ago? She and I used to take dance class together.

"Shelia, how are you? You look exactly the same."

Shelia smiled and said, "I'm fine. It's good to see you again."

They chatted for a few more minutes, and the woman and her husband trotted off to do more shopping. As the couple disappeared into the hardware section, Shelia looked at me, eyes wide, and confessed, "I have no idea who that woman was. I have no memory of ever knowing her." She paused and then said, "Get the expensive vacuum cleaner."

Having the proper balance of dietary healthy fats can make an enormous difference in mental, cardiovascular, immune, and neuronal health. Eating healthy foods helps keep these fats in the proper proportions.

There has been a lot of press about omega-3 and omega-6 fats. Both are essential fatty acids and necessary for good health. Unfortunately, for most of us the balance or the ratio of these fats is way off. Instead of being at the optimal omega-6 to omega-3 ratio of 1 to 1, the Western diet ratio is approximately 16 to 1. This means we are eating too many foods high in omega-6 fats and not enough foods high in omega-3s. What we want to do is get back in balance by eating more foods high in omega-3s, such as fish, soy, canola oil, vegetables, whole grains, nuts, and seeds, instead of foods that are highly processed, like commercial snack foods, baked goods, and frozen foods (not that all frozen foods are bad—plain frozen fruits and vegetables, with no added sauces, are terrific).

The high prevalence of omega-6 fats in our diet comes primarily from fast foods and processed foods high in vegetable oils, such as corn, cottonseed, soybean, and safflower, as well as from red meat. Omega-6 and omega-3 fatty acids (and omega-9s) are often found together naturally in foods. It is the overconsumption of meat and the processed and convenience foods that causes the problem. This is not to say that, for example, soybean or corn oil is bad for you. But these oils are used in processed foods, and we eat so much processed food and so little whole healthy food that the omega-3 and omega-6 balance is knocked off.

When the omega-6 and omega-3 balance is off, there is an increase in internal inflammation. Inflammation is the jumping-off point for many of the chronic diseases that plague us today. With too many omega-6s and not enough omega-3s, the body overproduces chemicals called eicosanoids. The kinds of eicosanoids that omega-6s produce are released in the body in response to injury, infection, stress, or certain diseases and thus are involved in the inflammation process. The omega-6-produced eicosanoids are important, but too many of them being dumped into the body for too long can create problems. Omega-3s, however, produce different kinds of eicosanoids that modify and reduce the omega-6s' inflammatory chemicals. When inflammation is ongoing, it becomes a bad thing instead of a healing process. For example, when you scrape your knee, it gets red and swollen. If you kept reinjuring that scrape, it would get very inflamed, oozy, and painful. After a while the inflammatory process would start to go awry, and the cut would get all mucked up. Your knee would become very painful. But when inflammation happens in your brain, neurons, or arteries, you do not feel anything. When it happens in your joints, you'll feel it eventually (for example, arthritis), but only after some damage has occurred. Eating whole, fresh foods and fewer processed foods and less red meat will help you regain the balance of omega-3s and omega-6s. Choose real potatoes instead of frozen french-fried potatoes (use olive oil, roasted garlic, or salsa as a topping instead of butter); baked chips instead of fried; broiled fish instead of a fried fish sandwich; and fresh frozen spinach instead of frozen creamed spinach.

I bought the expensive vacuum cleaner because it seemed awfully important to Shelia at that moment. Meanwhile, Shelia, who already ate pretty well and exercised regularly, made a concerted effort to increase her intake of omega-3 fatty acids from food and eat fewer processed foods. She also started taking omega-3 supplements. That was about a year ago, and though Shelia still does not remember who the mall woman was, she does say she feels her memory and mental clarity have improved.

Too many omega-6s from processed and convenience foods and red meat increase inflammation and the risk of brain farts and chronic diseases. Eat more omega-3s in whole, fresh foods like broccoli, oatmeal, walnuts, tofu, and flaxseed oil and skip the processed, packaged, pre-prepared foods as much as possible.

## Mood, Behavior, and Fats

As far as our brain goes, one of the distinguishing characteristics of Alzheimer's disease is inflammation. Studies are suggesting that anti-inflammatory agents such as NSAIDs (nonsteroidal anti-inflammatory drugs) are associated with a decreased risk of Alzheimer's disease. There is also some evidence to suggest that eating healthy unsaturated fats may reduce cognitive decline as we age.

The modern Western diet does not have enough essential fatty acids and has too much bad fat (saturated and trans). A disturbing finding in research is indicating that the *under*consumption of healthy fats like omega-3s parallels the rise in psychiatric disorders in recent years. Because of the way we eat and live, we are increasing our risk of cognitive decline. Marcy, a nutrition student of mine, told me her 12-year-old daughter had just had her tonsils out and was home recovering. "I am in charge of everything she has been eating and I can see a difference, a huge improvement in her mood, attitude, behavior, everything!" she said. "She's eating all healthy foods now. None of the junk or sweets she can get at school or with her friends." While her conclusion was not the result of a scientific study, it is not unusual to see an improvement in mood and behavior as a result of a better diet. When kids and adults alike clean up their diet and reduce their intake of bad fats, their brain gets healthier.

As if heart disease and obesity aren't bad enough, all the processed food, fast food, junk, sodas, and sweets we eat seem to contribute to depression and other mental disorders in children and adults.

Essential fatty acids (good fats) are critical components of neural membranes in our brain and nervous system. A paucity of good fats and an abundance of bad fats can compromise the ability of neurons to communicate and the generation of other brain and nervous system chemicals that regulate mood and behavior. Unsaturated fats lower cholesterol levels and thus help keep those tiny arteries in the head un-clogged. It would stand to reason that a diet high in anti-inflammatory foods with a balance of omega-3s and omega-6s would help decrease internal inflammation and possibly reduce the risk or magnitude of cognitive decline and dementias and improve symptoms of depression and other psychiatric illnesses.

Back in 1997 a high school for disruptive, at-risk students in Appleton, Wisconsin, began a very interesting journey. Over a period of a few years the school revamped its food program, adding a real kitchen to the premises, getting rid of junk food and replacing it with healthy foods and meals, and offering nutrition and physical education programs. You can guess what happened. No, the students did not protest the healthy changes. A report titled "Better Food, Better Behavior" found that not only did the Appleton students embrace the changes (with minor grumbling) but their concentration, schoolwork, and disruptive behavior all improved.

A study in 2002 in the *British Journal of Psychiatry* found that prisoners given supplements that included vitamins, minerals, and healthy fats had a "remarkable" reduction in antisocial behavior including violence. The Appleton students and the prisoners reportedly received tremendous benefits in behavior and mood from adding healthy fats and healthy foods to their diets. This isn't rocket science. The foods we choose to eat or give our kids have an impact on brain health, so it stands to reason that mood and behavior would be affected as well.

---

Bad fats and a lack of healthy omega-3s interfere with the brain's ability to function, which in turn affects mood and behavior.

---

## Babies

Fetuses' and babies' brains, nervous systems, and eyes need essential fatty acids for proper growth and development. The fetus and placenta are entirely dependent on maternal essential fatty acids for their supply. Studies are showing that fetuses and babies whose mothers are not eating enough healthy fats may suffer from neurological problems. But if you are pregnant, talk to your ob-gyn before you start taking omega-3 supplements. Skip the fast food, cheese, fried foods, sodas, and snack foods. Instead, eat more salads, chicken, fish, vegetables and fruits, and even peanut butter and jelly on whole-wheat bread with a glass of fat-free milk. Healthy foods will help you get the essential fatty acids you and the baby need. Be sure to scrupulously avoid any foods that have trans fats or hydrogenated oils.

---

Before and during pregnancy, be sure to eat an abundance of healthy fats from nuts, seeds, low-mercury fish, green vegetables, whole-grain breads and pastas, and fat-free milk, cheese, and yogurt.

---

## Dazed and Confused

You will hear about different omega-3 fatty acids (the difference lies in their molecular structure) and how some forms of these fats are better for you than others. DHA and EPA are the omega-3 fats of choice. Fish such as salmon, mackerel, sardines, flounder, and halibut are all good sources of omega-3 fatty acids.

In the plant world flaxseed oil, ground flaxseeds, walnuts, soy foods, seaweed, and canola oils are good sources of omega-3 fats, but they have a different form of omega-3 fats than fish do. Fish omega-3s and plant omegas-3s are kissing cousins, not identical twins.

There is an ongoing controversy about the extent of the benefits of the plant form of omega-3 fats, as some scientists say the body does not utilize this form well. Others disagree and say that for non–fish eaters upping the intake of plant foods high in omega-3s will help the body get back into omega balance and derive all the benefits thereof. If you do not eat fish, go for the omega-3 plant foods. Add some flaxseed oil to your salad, ground flaxseeds to your cereal or salad, edamame (green soybeans) to your pasta sauce, use canola oil instead of corn oil, throw some walnuts in your nonfat yogurt.

The omega-3 fat in fish is different from the omega-3 fats in plant foods like soy and walnuts. Just as jazz and R&B are different forms of music, the omega-3 fats in fish and those in plant foods are different forms of this essential fatty acid, and both are good for you.

## Benefits of Omega-3 Fats

Omega-3 Fats and Depression, Cognitive Decline, Alzheimer's Disease and Other Forms of Dementia

Could the solution to a moody child, depressed teen, or irritable grown-up be as simple as increasing their intake of omega-3 fats? Researchers cannot give us definitive answers yet, but studies are suggesting some possible connections:

- Major depression is associated with lowered omega-3 fatty acid levels.
- Low omega-3 levels may be associated with suicide attempts.
- Omega-3 fats may be helpful in treating or reducing depression in children and adults.
- Omega-3 fats are a critical part of brain and nervous system development in growing fetuses and babies.
- There may be an association between omega-3 fatty acids and reduced risk of dementia.
- Omega-3s may reduce brain inflammation and have a role in the regeneration of nerve cells.
- Dietary deficiency of omega-3s has been associated with schizophrenia.

## Omega-3s and Cardiovascular Disease

- Omega-3s reduce serum triglycerides (the fat floating in your blood, especially after a meal).
- The consumption of fish or fish oil (omega-3 fats) lowers risk of death from coronary heart disease, nonsudden death from a myocardial infarction (heart attack), and sudden death.
- Omega-3 fats help to keep blood clots from forming and may prevent cardiac arrhythmias.
- Omega-3 fatty acids may be protective against stroke.

## Other Omega-3 Benefits

- Evidence suggests that omega-3 fatty acids reduce tender joint pain for people suffering with rheumatoid arthritis.
- Omega-3 fats act as systemic anti-inflammatories.
- A diet rich in omega-3 fatty acids might help treat people with lung diseases such as asthma and emphysema.
- Plant sources of omega-3s, such as walnuts and flaxseeds, help keep bones strong and healthy.

# Healthy Fat Food Ideas

### BREAKFAST

Whole-grain cereal with ground flaxseeds,
fruit (½ banana or berries), nonfat milk
Coffee (use nonfat milk or a soy creamer), tea, fat-free milk, or
6 ounces of fresh 100 percent juice

### LUNCH

Hummus, chopped onions, tomatoes,
lettuce in whole-wheat pita with tahini and hot sauce (if you like it)
Tea, water, seltzer, or diet soda (if you must)

### SNACK #1 — *if you are a little hungry*

10 walnuts in 6 ounces nonfat yogurt
Tea or skim hot chocolate (no whip)

### SNACK #2 — *if you just feel like munching*

One snack bag of baked chips or tortilla chips
(with no trans fats or palm oil), salsa

### DINNER

Grilled fish
Spinach sautéed with garlic and olive oil
Whole-wheat couscous, steamed with ginger, cinnamon,
ground cumin

*Dessert*
Sorbet or fat-free frozen yogurt with berries
*Or*
A piece (not a chunk) of dark chocolate

Nothing suggests that omega-3 fatty acids will turn you into a rock star. But you never know!

## Omega-3s: To Supplement or Not to Supplement

Do not start taking omega-3 fish oil supplements or give them to your children without first discussing this with your health care practitioner. Though the research regarding supplementation and its health benefits is very compelling, there can be a down side too. Any supplement—vitamins, minerals, antioxidants, herbs, or fatty acids—can interact with medications or worsen certain conditions.

People taking more than 3 grams of omega-3 fatty acids from capsules should do so only under a physician's care. High intakes could cause excessive bleeding in some people.

---

**American Heart Association:**
**Summary of Recommendations for Omega-3 Fatty Acid Intake**

| Population | Recommendation |
| --- | --- |
| Patients without documented coronary heart disease (CHD) | Eat a variety of (preferably fatty) fish at least twice a week. Include oils and foods rich in alphalinolenic acid (flaxseed, canola, and soybean oils; flaxseed and walnuts). |
| Patients with documented CHD | Consume about 1 g of EPA+DHA per day, preferably from fatty fish. EPA+DHA in capsule form could be considered in consultation with the physician. |
| Patients who need to lower triglycerides | 2 to 4 grams of EPA+DHA per day provided as capsules under a physician's care. |

---

Source: "Fish and Omega-3 Fatty Acids," AHA Recommendations, 2006, www.americanheart.org/presenter.jhtml?identifier=4632.

### American Heart Association: For Women

As an adjunct to diet, omega-3 fatty acids in capsule form (approximately 850 to 1,000 mg of EPA and DHA) may be considered in women with CHD, and higher doses (2 to 4 grams) may be used for treatment of women with high triglyceride levels.

## Something's Fishy

There is a growing controversy about whether to eat fish or not. Here are the pros and cons of eating fish. Ultimately, the decision is up to you.

**Arguments *for* Eating Fish**
- Fish is an excellent source of omega-3 fatty acids EPA and DHA.
- Fish is an excellent source of lean, healthy protein.
- Diets high in fish are heart healthy.
- Eating broiled or baked fish is associated with lower risk of ischemic stroke (eating fried fish or fish sandwiches is associated with higher risk).
- Experts say the benefits of eating fish outweigh the potential risks.
- Fish consumption may slow cognitive decline.
- There is a good variety of fish.
- Fish is affordable for most people.
- If you do eat fish, the Environmental Defense Fund has information on low-mercury, low-pesticide fish that are not endangered: www.edf.org/page.cfm?tagID=1521

**Arguments *against* Eating Fish**
- Wild fish contain varying levels of methylmercury, which is a potent neurotoxin for fetuses, children, and adults.
- The 1999–2000 NHANES survey found that more than 300,000 newborns each year in the United States may have been exposed in utero to higher than acceptable methylmercury concentrations and may be at increased risk of adverse neurodevelopmental effects associated with methylmercury exposure.
- Farmed and wild fish contain varying amounts of PCBs (polychlorinated biphenyls), DDT, and dioxins, all of which are powerful poisons.
- Fish and shellfish contain heavy metals, organochlorine pesticides, and environmental contaminants.
- According to the UN Food and Agriculture Organization (FAO), 75 percent of the world's marine fish populations are fully fished, overfished, or depleted.

### What If You Are Pregnant?

The American Heart Association recommends that pregnant and lactating women

- avoid eating fish high in methylmercury (e.g., shark, swordfish, king mackerel, or tile fish);
- eat up to 12 ounces a week of a variety of fish and shellfish low in mercury; and
- check the Environmental Protection Agency and the U.S. Food and Drug Administration's Web sites for updates and local advisories about safety of local catch.

### What If You Don't Eat Fish?

- Non–fish eaters can get their omega-3 fatty acids from a diet high in foods such as ground flaxseeds, flaxseed oil, soy, tofu, canola oil, walnuts, walnut oil, and seaweed.
- Consider taking a daily algae-based DHA supplement providing 0.1 to 0.3 grams per capsule.
- Choose liquid oils and foods (e.g., flaxseed, walnuts, soybeans) that provide relatively high amounts of non-marine-derived omega-3 fatty acids.
- Consuming 1 ounce of walnuts or 1½ tablespoons of ground flaxseed would provide an amount of plant-derived omega-3 fatty acids in keeping with the recommendations from the Institute of Medicine.
- Avoid foods high in omega-6 fatty acids, such as processed and convenience foods and red meat.

## Saturated Fat

Animal foods contain a kind of fat called saturated fat (the word *saturated* has to do with its chemical structure). Saturated fat is found primarily in animal foods. The only exceptions to this are the tropical oils—coconut, palm, and palm kernel—and cocoa butter, which come from plant sources. These are also saturated. In the United States tropical oils are found mostly in processed foods such as commercially

---

### The Naked Truth

*There is no fat that is 100 percent saturated or unsaturated. Most fats contain both saturated and unsaturated fatty acids. The fats that are mostly chemically saturated are classified as such, and the same goes for unsaturated fats. For example, canola oil, an unsaturated fat, is about 7 percent saturated, with the rest being unsaturated, and it is liquid at room temperature. Compare that with butter, a saturated fat, which is 60 percent saturated and solid at room temperature, and you can see why they are classified differently.*

---

produced cakes, cookies, margarines, crackers, and candy bars. Unlike *un*saturated fats, saturated fats are solid at room temperature, like butter, cheese (ALL kinds of cheese), lard, bacon fat, milk fat, and the fat in beef, ham, bologna, pork, and lamb.

For some reason people always tell me they don't eat a lot of fat or a lot of food. When Bill came to see me, he was obese and had undergone a procedure called a cardiac catheterization. A "cath" is a diagnostic procedure in which a thin plastic tube is inserted into an artery or vein and snaked up until it reaches the heart. The results indicated that he had arterial blockages and was at risk of a heart attack.

Bill worked in the music business, traveled a lot, entertained often, and was a self-described "foodie." Bill loved good food and cooking gourmet meals for his friends. When I asked him to give me a sample of what he ate in a day, his choices included cheese, osso buco, roasted veal, baked brie, flan, and bread and butter. All these foods are laden with saturated fat and very high in calories. Bill was going to have to make some big changes in his lifestyle if he wanted to lower his risk of having a heart attack.

All saturated fats when eaten regularly—daily or several times a week—can make you sick. The reason is that saturated fat has a chemical reaction in the body that increases internal inflammation, serum cholesterol, LDL cholesterol (the bad cholesterol), and arterial inflammation and dysfunction. Saturated fat has also been associated with an increased risk of atherosclerosis and diabetes and may increase fat storage in your abdomen (commonly referred to as ab flab). Ab flab in and of itself increases the risk of heart disease and diabetes. Studies have shown that eating red meat, a significant source of bad saturated fat, may increase the risk of colorectal cancer and lung cancer (irrespective of smoking status), and some experts believe red meat may be linked to prostate cancer. In 2009 a study of over half a million people found a link between eating red meat and a greater risk of death from cancer and cardiovascular disease. Red meat includes steak and veal, and processed meats include hot dogs, bologna, salami, and sausage. In comparison, the study found reduced risks of cancer and heart disease deaths in people who ate white meat (such as chicken breast) and fish. To date this is the largest study of its kind. Scientists are not sure whether the increased cancer and cardiovascular disease risk among meat eaters is due to the saturated fat, the way the meat is processed, or some other variables they have not yet identified.

---

Saturated fat comes mostly from animals. Any food that comes from an animal, such as beef, pork, salami, lamb, bacon, milk, cheese, and butter, has saturated fat. Saturated fat does bad things inside the body every time you eat it. Eating foods that contain this bad fat every day over a period of weeks and years increases the risk of a lot of very unpleasant diseases. A little bit of saturated fat (16–20 grams) each day is OK, but most people eat a lot more than that.

---

## How Does Saturated Fat Affect the Brain?

Imagine how small the arteries in your brain are. Now imagine even the tiniest bit of arterial plaque in those teeny arteries and how that could impede blood flow and oxygen delivery to the brain. The inflammation caused by the saturated fat we eat, the increase in serum cholesterol (cholesterol floating in the blood) and LDL (bad) cholesterol caused by dietary saturated fat, creates the formation of the gunk that clogs up arteries. Even a small loss of blood flow to your brain can cause problems. A small study in the *Journal of the American College of Cardiology* in 2006 found that a single meal high in saturated fat (e.g., a cheeseburger) can impair blood vessel function and decrease anti-inflammatory action of HDL (good) cholesterol. Another clinical study, in the journal *Arteriosclerosis, Thrombosis & Vascular Biology*, discovered that after only three weeks those subjects who ate a high saturated-fat diet suffered from a 50 percent decrease in their arteries' ability to dilate to accommodate blood flow. Imagine what eating burgers, bacon, steak, cheese, and ice cream does to your blood vessels if eaten several times a week or more.

Gunked-up arteries, also known as cardiovascular disease, restrict blood flow and limit the delivery of oxygen and other life-sustaining compounds to every organ in the body. Elevated cholesterol levels have been associated with amyloid plaques in the brain. Amyloid plaques are a buildup and hardening of protein fragments in the brain and are thought to be a hallmark of Alzheimer's disease. Aside from the obvious heart disease, stroke, and high blood pressure that cardiovascular disease lends itself to, current research has found that cardiovascular disease may lead to a decline in cognitive function and an increased risk of dementia and Alzheimer's disease. Additionally, as research continues, findings are pointing toward a relationship between dietary saturated fats, the incidence of Alzheimer's disease, and an increased decline in cognitive function. In Finland, a study of more than 1,500 people found that eating a lot of saturated fat in midlife increased the risk of cognitive decline later in life. Eating good unsaturated fats was associated with better memory and overall cognitive function later on in life.

If you eat foods that contain saturated fat, such as ham and ice cream, you may be contributing to clogged arteries and inflammation in your brain. You may even be increasing the risk of developing dementia or cognitive decline. What you eat now will affect your health later.

**Saturated Surprises**

| Food | Saturated Fat (in grams) |
| --- | --- |
| M&M® McFlurry® (12-fluid-oz cup) | 12 |
| Au Bon Pain plain croissant | 9 |
| KFC Chicken Pot Pie | 31 |
| 6 oz meat loaf | 10.6 |
| 2 slices (2 oz) cheddar cheese | 6 |
| 1 boneless broiled pork chop | 5.4 |

Sources: www.nutrition.mcdonalds.com/nutritionexchange/nutrition_facts.html; www.aubonpain.
com/menu/food.aspx?s=cafe_bakery&f=17; www.kfc.com/nutrition/pdf/kfc_nutrition_april09.pdf;
USDA National Nutrient Database for Standard Reference, Release 21, U.S. Department of Agriculture,
Agricultural Research Service, 2009, www.ars.usda.gov/ba/bhnrc/ndl.

☞   Saturated fat is a bad fat.

☞   Saturated fat is found primarily in foods that come from ani-
      mals, such as beef, lamb, pork, ham, milk, cheese, and butter.

☞   Plant sources of saturated fat are coconut, palm, and palm kernel
      oils.

☞   Saturated fat raises LDL cholesterol (the bad cholesterol).

☞   Nonfat or low-fat versions of animal foods, such as nonfat milk,
      cheese, yogurt, or light or low-fat mayo, are OK to eat.

☞   Saturated fat increases internal inflammation, cholesterol, and
      the risk of heart disease, cancer, diabetes, Alzheimer's disease,
      and other forms of dementia.

Remember our friend Bill? He stuck with the program. Came to nutrition classes and counselings. Began a regular exercise routine. In three
months he had lost 20 pounds. "I feel better than I have ever felt in
my life," Bill admitted. "And there is something else. I used to feel
overwhelmed by all the paperwork I had to do, and now it seems so
much more manageable. I feel like my mind went through the car wash."
About six months later Bill came back for a visit to show off his new

> *The Nurses' Health Study is an ongoing study that began in 1976 when 121,700 female registered nurses ages 30 to 55 completed a medical history and health-related behaviors questionnaire. Since then, the women have completed questionnaires about every two years. Researchers have discovered volumes of essential information about lifestyle, nutrition behaviors, and their relation to disease risk. In 2007 the Nurses' Health Study found that women who ate diets high in animal, saturated, and trans fats were more likely to gain weight.*

**Kid Fact:** Children under the age of 2 can consume whole milk and dairy products. After the age of 2 they should go low-fat or nonfat with milk, cheese, ice cream, and all other foods that come from animals.

and improved physique. He had lost an additional 30 pounds. "Can you keep it up?" I asked. "Yes," Bill said. "I can. This was a total lifestyle change. I still love food and eating out and entertaining, I just do it differently now. I never want to have to be cathed again, that's for sure."

Adopting a healthy lifestyle that includes a substantial reduction in eating foods that contain saturated fat—foods from animals—may prevent the majority of cardiovascular disease in Western populations. As much as you love your butter, burgers, and brisket, your brain, heart, and arteries do not. Reducing the intake of saturated fat can significantly decrease cholesterol levels, which means less internal inflammation and less of a chance of clogging those minuscule arteries in your head. For an easy first step to reducing saturated fat, go low-fat or non-fat with all dairy foods. Eating nonfat milk, cheese, yogurt, and ice cream can really help lower the amount of saturated fat you eat every day. There are some pretty decent low-fat or nonfat cheeses around—for example, part-skim mozzarella. And forget about using butter, which is just a stick of saturated fat. Find margarines that have no hydrogenated oils and little or no palm or coconut oils. No matter what the front of the package says, the only way to know what is in the food product you are buying is to read the ingredient list. Yes, you have to read the microscopic print on the label, so bring your glasses.

## What to Do

- Choose low-fat or nonfat animal foods, including fat-free milk, cheese, and cottage cheese, white-meat poultry without skin (dark meat has more bad fat than the white meat), fish, and egg whites.
- Try alternatives to animal protein like soy, nuts, legumes (beans), and seeds.
- Indulge in "regular" fatty animal foods only on rare occasions. Rare means once or twice a month—not three or four times a week.
- Use plant fats (oils) to replace animal fats—for example, olive oil, canola oil, or nonhydrogenated margarine instead of butter.

As you well know, cognitive decline is not limited to older folks. I was doing some work in a nursing home and saw a relatively young woman on the dementia unit I had not seen before. I thought she was visiting a family member. Then she started saying, "Is this mine? Is this mine or yours? Is this mine?" over and over again. I looked at the nurse, silently questioning her. The nurse said quietly, "She's a new resident. Those are the only words she can say. She is in her early fifties." Sometimes genetics or other factors over which we have no control take hold of our brain. The best we can do is do the best we can, and that includes making healthy lifestyle choices. Diseases that are mostly preventable, such as obesity, cardiovascular disease, diabetes, and high blood pressure, may predispose people of any age to cognitive decline and Alzheimer's disease. With the increase in the prevalence of all these diseases in younger people, it is fair to say that entire generations may be at high risk of losing brain power earlier and suffering serious cognitive problems at younger ages.

**Ham Fact:** One typical ham and Swiss cheese sandwich can set you back about 13 grams of saturated fat. That is almost a whole day's worth of artery-clogging fat. How do you make it better? Use fat-free low-sodium ham—even better, choose grilled chicken breast and low-fat cheese on whole-grain bread with mustard. Easy.

To reduce the risk of chronic disease and brain decline, people of all ages need to make some serious dietary and lifestyle changes. Eating poorly, not exercising, and being overweight are likely to get a whole generation sicker and losing brain power at younger ages.

The bottom line is that our bodies were designed to tolerate only a small amount of daily dietary saturated fat. In our fast-food-, meat-, and cheese-soaked culture we are eating far too much saturated fat and are getting sick because of it. The American Heart Association recommends that 7 percent of calories per day come from saturated fat. But who knows how many calories they are eating every day (let alone who would take the time to calculate 7 percent of them)? A general recommendation is to limit your intake to about 16–20 grams of saturated fat or less per day. Unlike with essential fatty acids, you do not need to eat saturated fat in order to be healthy. The easiest way to limit saturated fat is to drastically reduce your consumption of animal foods unless they are low-fat or nonfat choices. Low-fat or nonfat means that much

### Get Smart's Nutrition Prescription for Healthy Fats

| Instead of | Choose |
| --- | --- |
| Cream cheese | Fat-free cream cheese or tofu cream cheese |
| Butter | Peanut butter |
| Butter | Vegan margarine (e.g., Earth Balance; it has about half the saturated fat of butter) |
| Regular cheeses | Fat-free American, cheddar, Swiss, mozzarella cheeses (these make great grilled cheese sandwiches) |
| Drumstick | Grilled chicken breast, no skin |
| Whole or 2% milk | Fat-free or 1% milk |
| Regular omelet with cheese | Egg white omelet with fat-free cheese |
| Regular mayo | Fat-free or light mayo |
| Beef, veal, lamb | Grilled salmon, tilapia, or sole |
| Meat sauce, Alfredo sauce | Marinara or primavera sauces |
| Cheese and pepperoni pizza | Pizza with lots of vegetables and fat-free or part-skim mozzarella |
| Beef meatballs | Turkey meatballs |
| Ice cream | Fat-free frozen yogurt |
| Store-bought cookies | Homemade cookies |

or all of the bad fat has been removed from that food product. This is true for both saturated and trans fats. White-meat chicken, fish, fat-free milk and yogurt, and low-fat cream cheese are good choices.

---

Eating foods such as nonfat milk, yogurt, and cheese can help you reduce your intake of saturated fats. Sticking to white-meat chicken and turkey, fish, and egg whites as the main animal protein in your diet will help enormously too. Focus on choosing more plant foods like beans, nuts, seeds, and soy in place of animal foods. Have vegetarian chili, hummus dip and vegetables, a grilled nonfat cheese and tomato sandwich, pizza with part-skim mozzarella and lots of vegetables, or a grilled tofu stir fry.

---

## Trans Fats

In 1902 when trans fats were invented in a new chemical process in Germany called hydrogenation, a whole new era in food production began. These new artificially produced fats could be used in place of butter and lard, fried at high temperatures without burning, increase the shelf life of foods, and add important textures to foods like "crispy" and "flaky." Hydrogenation turns an oil, which is liquid at room temperature, into a solid. Take corn oil, for instance. On the supermarket shelf it is a golden liquid. But heat it up and add some chemicals, and voila, you've got a hard stick of corn oil margarine. Food companies caught on and began using trans fats in commercially produced baked goods—like cookies, coffee cakes, muffins, pie crusts, and crackers—candy, and frozen foods. The creamy center in the original Oreo cookie was made of whipped lard. When lard started getting bad press because it is a saturated fat and trans fats hit the commercial market, the Oreo people started using trans fats instead of lard to make the white stuff. Restaurants and fast-food chains started using trans fats exclusively for deep frying foods like french fries, tempura, fried chicken, calamari, shrimp, and onions. Doughnuts are fried in vats of trans fats (though some of the bigger doughnut chains have recently stopped using trans fats).

Artificially produced trans fats are unhealthy. There are some trans fats found in nature, but not many. Artificially produced trans fats are found in store-bought foods like cookies, cakes, crackers, snacks, and frozen foods as well as fried foods in most restaurants.

## Fast-forward a Few Decades

Research can be tedious and sometimes lag behind the times. But in the case of trans fats, researchers began to catch on relatively quickly just how bad these fake fats are. Back in 1956 in an editorial in the medical journal the *Lancet*, one scientist speculated that trans fats might increase the risk of cardiovascular disease. Still, it took a while before trans fats got some press. In 1990 a study found that trans fats lowered good cholesterol (HDL) and raised bad cholesterol (LDL). In 1994 researchers at the Harvard School of Public Health reported that more than "30,000 deaths per year may be due to consumption of partially hydrogenated vegetable fat. Furthermore, the number of attributable cases of nonfatal coronary heart disease will be even larger." In 2006 these researchers revised their estimate, suggesting that up to 228,000 coronary heart disease events could be *avoided* by the reduction or elimination of trans fats from the American diet.

The wheels of change are slow, and it was not until early in the twenty-first century that food companies began removing trans fats from their products. In 2003 Stephen Jacobs, a cookie consumer and lawyer in San Francisco, began a lawsuit against the Kraft Company alleging that Oreos were unhealthy because of the trans fat. This generated a lot of media attention, and people started becoming more aware of the dangers of trans fats. The lawsuit was dropped when Kraft dropped the trans fat from the Oreos. Some U.S. cities and states are beginning to ban the use of trans fats in restaurants, but they are still found in many commercially prepared foods.

Trans fats are really bad for you. Drastically reducing or eliminating trans fats from your diet may just save your life. And your kids' lives.

## What's the Dish?

If you can believe it, trans fats are even worse than saturated fats. They not only increase LDL cholesterol (the bad cholesterol) but also lower HDL cholesterol (the good cholesterol), increase the risk of diabetes, gall stones, and internal inflammation, and may have deleterious effects on babies in the womb when eaten in quantity by the mother. In the brain and other neurons in the body trans fats may become incorporated into cell membranes and impair their ability to function, communicate, and transport nutrients. Trans fats are just close enough in structure to healthy fats to stand in for them in biological functions. But they cannot do the job of the healthy fats and so cause dysfunction and disease.

**Home Cooking Fact:** Sautéing or frying foods at home in healthy oils, like olive or canola oil, will not turn them into trans fats.

Trans fats contribute to a lot of diseases like heart disease, diabetes, infertility, and neurological problems in growing fetuses.

☞ Artificially produced trans fats are bad.

☞ Trans fats are in processed foods like cookies, crackers, snack foods, and margarine.

☞ Most deep fried foods in restaurants, such as french fries, fried chicken, tempura, and doughnuts, are fried in trans fats (except in states where trans fats are banned).

☞ Trans fats increase the risk of heart disease, sudden death, and diabetes.

☞ Trans fats may increase the risk of Alzheimer's disease and cognitive decline.

☞ Trans fats eaten by pregnant women may have detrimental effects on the neurological conditions of their babies. In other words, if you are pregnant, avoid eating foods that contain trans fatty acids (hydrogenated oils).

☞ Trans fats can become incorporated into neurons in the brain and interfere with their function.

☞ Trans fats may increase the risk of ovulatory infertility.

## The Trans Fat Trap

There is no definitive recommendation for how much trans fats one can consume daily because there is nothing healthy about them. Public policy is catching up, and trans fats are being used less and less in processed foods and restaurants, but it is up to you to check whether the foods you eat have trans fats. Your best bet is to avoid them as much as possible. Look for the words *partially hydrogenated* in the ingredient list on food labels. Even when a product says "No Trans Fats," it can contain as much as 0.5 gram or less per serving.

## Cholesterol

**Cognitive Decline Fact:** Diabetes, high blood pressure, obesity, metabolic syndrome, and cardiovascular disease are associated with the risk of cognitive decline and in some cases Alzheimer's disease and other forms of dementia.

Cholesterol has gotten such a bad rap. It is blamed for the more than 80 million cases of cardiovascular disease in the United States. And yet cholesterol, another kind of fat, is an essential part of every cell membrane in the body, the central nervous system, hormones, and other physiological functions. In fact, cholesterol is so important to the health of the human body that it is made inside the body. Your liver makes cholesterol and sends it out into the bloodstream for your body to use. Since the liver makes cholesterol and plants do not have livers, you can assume that cholesterol is found only in animal foods. And since the liver makes cholesterol, we do not need to eat it to supply our bodies with the cholesterol they need.

Cholesterol is found only in foods that come from animals. Contrary to common belief, peanut butter does not contain cholesterol. Cholesterol is made inside your body by the liver and is necessary for a healthy brain and body.

There is good cholesterol (HDL), bad cholesterol (LDL), and other kinds of cholesterol that we need not delve into. The biochemistry is very complicated (and you were so sure that as an electrician, dancer, mechanic, stock broker, real estate agent, mother, or musician you would *never* need chemistry). The LDL's job is to deliver cholesterol to the cells. When there is too much LDL cholesterol circulating in the bloodstream (like after eating a cheeseburger, steak, or milkshake), it can cause inflammation in the lining of the artery. Over time the results of this inflammatory process cause glop (aka plaque) to build up and begin to clog the arteries. Plaque and sometimes blood clots form. Both can block arteries, causing a heart attack or stroke. HDL cholesterol is cardio-protective and helps reduce inflammation and plaque buildup in the arteries. This is why you hear so much about wanting a low LDL cholesterol and a high HDL cholesterol.

Both LDL (bad) and HDL (good) cholesterol are needed in the body. HDL cholesterol cleans up excess LDL cholesterol and has anti-inflammatory actions. But when there is not enough HDL or there is too much LDL, the risk of jammed-up, irritated arteries increases.

- Cholesterol is important for a healthy body.
- Cholesterol is made in the liver and plays critical roles in the central nervous system, hormone production, brain health, and cell membranes.
- Good cholesterol (HDL) and bad cholesterol (LDL) need to be in balance.
- Cholesterol is found in foods from animals and usually hangs out with its cousin, saturated fat.
- It is a good idea to limit consumption of animal foods.

> *If you believe what you read on the Internet, coconut oil will protect*
> *you from heart disease, cancer, obesity, and infections. There is little or*
> *no scientific evidence to support these claims. In fact, ounce for ounce,*
> *coconut oil is more saturated than either butter or lard, and studies have*
> *found that it raises cholesterol. Since coconut oil is saturated, it is solid*
> *at room temperature and may be used to replace trans fats in processed*
> *foods. Experts say it is OK to use coconut occasionally but not on a*
> *daily basis. Coconut meat or milk can be used as a garnish, in cooking,*
> *or in a piña colada (don't forget the little umbrella).*

Though saturated fat and cholesterol are two very different kinds of fats, they are usually found together in animal foods. It is best to considerably reduce your intake of these foods.

### What about Eating Cholesterol-Rich Foods?

Egg yolks and shellfish are two notable examples of foods high in cholesterol but low in saturated fat. Some people are sensitive to the cholesterol found in the food they eat, and it can cause undesirable effects in the arteries. It is almost impossible to know whether you are one of these cholesterol-sensitive people, so it is a good idea not to eat too many egg yolks or too much shellfish each week.

The National Cholesterol Education Program recommends eating less than 200 milligrams (mg) a day of cholesterol. What does this mean in terms of real food? One egg yolk contains about 210 mg of cholesterol. One small broiled pork chop has 53 mg of cholesterol, and only 3 ounces (a few pieces) of broiled shrimp has 166 mg of cholesterol. You see it can add up quickly. Aim for two or fewer yolks per week, including yolks in baked goods and in cooked or processed foods.

### Big Surprise

A nurse once told me, "You know I don't exercise or watch what I eat. And look at me. I look good." Then there was my neighbor in New

York—a lovely, young, small, thin babe. When she walked—strutted, actually—down the street, all the men gaped at her. She thought that because she was thin (she did not eat much, but that is a whole other story), she did not need to exercise. Then there are the guys at the gym who work out, lift weights, and head out for a 4-pound burger, large fries, and a protein drink on their way home. They figure since they are pretty studly they can eat anything they want. This is a common misconception and, I would add, a fervent hope. Unfortunately, exercising or being thin, or both, does not undo the ill effects of bad fats on the brain or the cardiovascular system that nourishes the brain and the heart.

A case in point was Tony, a 43-year-old construction worker and amateur competitive swimmer. He was at the pool at 5:00 a.m. most days, training intensely for two hours before he went to his physically demanding job. One day, famished after an intense workout, he stopped on his way to work and ate five hot dogs. Later that morning he began experiencing chest pain and was rushed to the emergency room. He was having a heart attack. "I was shocked," Tony said. "Never in a million years did I think I would have a heart attack. I did not give a thought to what I ate because I was in good shape, at a good weight." After attending several nutrition classes and counseling sessions, Tony told me, "You know, I think those hot dogs saved my life. I now know that all that bad fat and sodium had a really bad effect on my arteries. Maybe if I had the heart attack later, it would have been worse." The moral of the story is that even if you are at a good weight and exercise, eating saturated fat (foods from animals, such as bacon, lard, and roast beef) and trans fats can still cause a lot of problems. Saturated and trans fats cause a chemical reaction in the body that raises the LDL (bad) cholesterol floating in the blood and causes inflammation inside the whole body. Being a healthy weight and working out are incredibly important to good health, but you still have to eat healthy fats and foods.

## What to Do

In addition to following *Get Smart*'s Nutrition Prescription for healthy fats, here are other things you should do:

- If you are diabetic: keep your blood glucose in control.

- If you have high blood pressure: limit sodium, eat a lot of vegetables (see online the DASH diet at http://dashdiet.org/).
- If you are overweight: see a registered dietitian to help you make a healthy weight loss plan.
- If you have cardiovascular disease: choose a heart healthy diet (*Get Smart*'s Nutrition Prescription Plan is heart healthy).
- If you have any of the above, even if you do not: exercise daily.

---

- **Fats from plants and fish are good for you and important for a healthy, well-functioning brain and body.**

- **Good fats include mono- and polyunsaturated oils like fish, olive, canola, walnut, flaxseed, sesame, and peanut oils.**

- **Fats from animals are not good for you and increase the risk of disease and mental decline.**

- **Bad fats are trans fatty acids and saturated fats.**

- **You can still eat out, have fun, and entertain while eating healthy fats.**

- **Eating saturated fat and cholesterol once in a while is OK.**

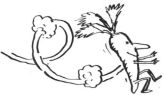

---

Margo will forgive you if you share your *Get Smart* Nutrition Prescription with her. Because, if you hadn't noticed, she forgot your name too.

# CHAPTER TWO

# Brain Spas: Protein

## KEY POINTS

⇨ The brain is able to perform 20 million billion calculations per second.

⇨ The brain needs a daily supply of amino acids to help perform these functions.

⇨ Protein is made up of amino acids.

⇨ Amino acids are necessary for healthy brain function.

⇨ Neurotransmitters are what the brain uses to send IMs.

⇨ Amino acids are the basis of many neurotransmitters.

⇨ Healthy protein comes from plants and animals.

—— NUTRITION PRESCRIPTION ——
*for* PROTEIN

⇨ **Have protein with breakfast.**

⇨ **Eat healthy protein with every meal and snack.**

⇨ **Acceptable animal proteins include fish, eggs, white-meat poultry, low-fat and nonfat dairy foods.**

⇨ **Focus on plant proteins such as soy, nuts, beans, and whole grains.**

A PIECE OF TOAST WITH butter. A blueberry muffin the size of a basketball. A bowl of sugar-frosted, honey-dipped, chocolate-coated cereal. These are typical breakfasts for many people as they dash out the door to start their day. Then midmorning hits, energy flags, thoughts are sluggish, and you stumble to the doughnut cart for a honey-glazed energy boost and your third 32-ounce cup of coffee with a shot of espresso. Aside from the lack of healthy carbohydrates (we'll cover that in the carbohydrate chapter), what is missing from these breakfasts is a nice protein bath. Your brain needs to be bathed in amino acids all day to facilitate its ability to perform the 20 million billion calculations per second of which it is capable. Generally we think of protein as a muscle-building nutrient, which it is, but protein is also intimately involved with brain function and total body health. Made up of amino acids, proteins participate in the immune system, hormone production, synaptic communication, and the structure and function of skin, bones, and organs. Amino acids, the building blocks of protein, are primarily what the brain uses to send billions of instant messages among neurons. There are 20 amino acids. Our bodies can make 10 of the necessary amino acids. The only way to get the other 10 amino acids is through the diet, by eating protein. These are called essential amino acids. How they line up, how long the string is, and what shape the string is (think of DNA's double helix) will determine their function. There are at least 10,000 different proteins in the human body.

You want your brain to be bathed in spa-quality proteins. Not the cheap and tawdry stuff but luxury high-end amino acids. In terms of diet there are two sources of protein: protein from animals and protein from plants. Healthy protein, the top-drawer quality, is lean and low in saturated (bad) fat. In the animal kingdom that includes fish, white-meat poultry, low-fat and nonfat diary foods, and egg whites. In the plant world protein is found in nuts, seeds, whole grains, beans, and vegetables. Animal protein that comes from red meat, whole milk and cheese, luncheon meats, deli meats, and ice cream is tied up with bad saturated fat. The protein itself is fine, but the package is what makes it bad. High-fat animal protein is the cheap and tawdry stuff, which is fun, but only on rare occasions. Stick with the top-drawer proteins for the majority of your brain baths.

Proteins play multiple roles in the body. Proteins are made up of different amino acids. Healthy sources of plant protein come from nuts, seeds, grains, beans, and vegetables. Healthy animal protein sources include egg whites (considered the "perfect" protein), white-meat poultry, fish, and low-fat and nonfat dairy foods like fat-free milk and cheese. Your brain uses amino acids to make the chemicals that send instant messages.

| The Cast of Amino Acids | | |
|---|---|---|
| Alanine | Glycine | Proline |
| Arginine | Histidine | Serine |
| Asparagine | Isoleucine | Threonine |
| Aspartic Acid | Leucine | Tryptophan |
| Cysteine | Lysine | Tyrosine |
| Glutamic Acid | Methionine | Valine |
| Glutamine | Phenylalanine | |

## Brain Texting

OMG. GR8 B%K. LOL. ☺

We communicate with each other by talking or texting, but the 100 billion neurons in your brain communicate with each other via electrical impulses and chemicals. The chemicals neurons use to communicate are called neurotransmitters. There are two groups of neurotransmitters that are made up of or derived from amino acids, and there is one group that comes from an essential nutrient called choline. Neurotransmitters affect mood, behavior, cognition, memory, arousal, movement, posture, appetite, pain, learning, heart rate, and many other functions.

Neurotransmitters are the chemical messengers your brain uses to send instant messages at lightning speed. Two groups of neurotransmitters are made up of amino acids, some of which we get through our diet and some of which our body makes. Neurotransmitters have a direct effect on mood and behavior.

## Bad Fad Diets

High-protein diets became very popular in the 1990s and early twenty-first century (one in particular, which shall remain nameless). They advocated eating bacon, beef, cheese, and butter and virtually eliminating carbohydrates from the diet. The high-protein, high-fat, low-carbohydrate fad diets to which I am referring caused a lot of controversy, and I was a vocal opponent of the diet for all the reasons stated in this book. High-fat animal foods increase the risk of dementia, heart disease, diabetes, obesity, and cancers. I had so many patients who were recovering from heart attacks who had been on one of these popular diets for the months preceding their cardiac event. Heart disease takes time to develop, so six months on this fad diet did not cause their disease, but it could have hastened the disease process.

In addition, as with all "diets," they do not work. Few people can stick to a "diet" for very long and are destined to regain any weight they may have lost. Diets mean deprivation and hunger, and some are quite expensive. They do not take into account life's realities. Nutrition Prescription for a Healthy Brain is about making healthy food choices that support healthy brain function. It's that simple.

The high-bad-fat, low-carb diets did have a silver lining. They highlighted the need to look at how protein affects weight loss and have sparked a host of scientific studies on the subject. Preliminary results have been interesting, suggesting that increasing healthy protein and reducing carbohydrates may facilitate weight loss and increase satiety (feeling satisfied after a meal). The operative word here is *healthy* protein. Not the high-fat protein the fad diets recommend. Since the effects of long-term higher-protein, low-carbohydrate diets remain unknown, it is best to focus on adopting a balanced, healthy eating plan first. Then deal with weight loss by eating less if that is the final goal.

---

Popular high-protein fad diets tend to be high in bad saturated fat and other bad foods. They can be expensive and are generally totally unrealistic for most of us. They are notoriously low in vegetables, fruits, beans, and other health-promoting foods. Increasing healthy protein like soy, nuts, and egg whites and cutting back on some carbohydrates like rice and bread may benefit your brain and your body.

---

☞ Popular high-protein fad diets contain a lot of bad saturated fat.

☞ Diets high in this bad inflammatory fat increase the risk of cardiovascular disease, diabetes, and dementia.

☞ Healthy protein in place of some (not all) carbohydrates may help with weight loss.

☞ Long-term effects of higher-protein diets are not yet known.

Anna had struggled with weight all her life. She showed me pictures of herself as a chubby 3-year-old. "My family is from Spain, and hot meals were an important part of family life," Anna told me. "My sister and I used to stay with my grandparents during the day, and they would give us snacks and a big hot meal midday. Then we'd go home, and our parents would give us more snacks and another big hot meal." At 48, Anna, a physician with a full-time job at a hospital and a growing family, was stunned to discover she had high cholesterol and high triglycerides and was heading into morbid obesity. "I was devastated," Anna said. She had tried every diet including high-protein, low-carbohydrate; liquid fasts; and premade frozen dinners, but nothing worked. She always regained any weight she lost. After seeing her blood test, Anna decided to take control. She started exercising two to three days a week with a certified trainer and keeping a food record (writing down everything she ate). After the first week she reviewed her food record. "I couldn't believe how much I was eating!" She cut out snacks such as pretzels and Goldfish, added more vegetables, and skipped desserts. In six months she had lost 22 pounds, and all her blood tests came back normal. She was thrilled. "I have only made a few, pretty easy changes in my diet and look at the results." To ensure her continued success Anna started seeing me and together we created a healthy eating plan that she and her family can live with. One big change we made was the addition of healthy protein, like egg whites or peanut butter, in every breakfast. "My kids and I feel like we are eating *real food* now," Anna said. "All of us have more energy in the mornings and I don't need to snack before lunch anymore."

## Daily Dose

The brain cannot store amino acids, so it needs an ongoing daily supply from the food we eat. Most Americans consume plenty of protein. Eating too little protein affects the health of your whole body, including the ability of the neurons in your brain to communicate. Having protein with every meal feeds your brain and helps increase satiety (feeling full), helps manage energy and blood sugar levels, may increase weight and fat loss, and may build muscles (technically only exercise "builds" muscles, but they won't get built without adequate dietary protein).

Think Goldilocks; not too much, not too little, but juuuust right. What that means is getting the right amount of protein in your meals. Go for serving sizes of 3–4 ounces of fish or poultry. Half a cup of cooked beans. Two tablespoons of peanut butter. Eight ounces of nonfat milk and yogurt. Replacing high-fat protein like cheese, beef, and lamb with low-fat protein like fat-free cheese, chicken, and tofu may help your brain and your waistline. A multiethnic study in Canada found that people who substituted a small amount of healthy protein (e.g., chicken or fish) for carbohydrates (bread, cookies) showed a reduction in their waistline. Instead of having a corn muffin the size of a Volkswagen for breakfast, have a whole-wheat English muffin with peanut butter.

### Protein: A multitasking nutrient

**Structural proteins:** *Just like the scaffold on a new building, some proteins serve as the structure upon which teeth, bones, and skin are built. They also are an integral part of your organs and muscles.*

**Fluid balance:** *Proteins help maintain the body's fluid balance.*

**Antibodies:** *Antibodies are large proteins that fight invasions of foreign substances like bacteria and viruses.*

**Hormones:** *Hormones act as messengers in the body, and many are made up of amino acids.*

**Transport proteins:** *Some proteins act like taxis carrying vitamins and other substances in the blood from place to place.*

**Enzymes:** *Proteins work to speed up certain chemical reactions in the body.*

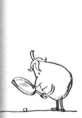

☞   The brain needs a regular supply of amino acids.

☞   We get amino acids from dietary protein.

☞   Protein is good to include with each meal and snack.

☞   Most Americans get enough protein in their diets.

## Neurotransmitters: The Stuff of Dreams

Otto Loewi, pharmacologist and physiologist, discovered the first neurotransmitter, acetylcholine, in 1921. Popular mythology says the idea for
the experiment that led to the discovery came to Dr. Loewi in a dream.
He won the Nobel Prize for his research in 1936. Understanding the
link between diet and neurotransmitters, the brain's chemical messengers, requires some explanation, so please bear with me. For most of us,
eating healthy sources of protein ensures that our brain gets the amino
acids it needs. Poor diet, stress, infection, and some medications can
deplete the levels of neurotransmitters in the brain. However, supple-
menting with specific amino acids, unless directed by your physician, is
not recommended. These substances are potent and play many different
roles in the body. Taking concentrated doses of any single amino acid
may cause problems. For example, tryptophan and tyrosine are common amino acids that have opposing effects in the brain. Tryptophan
calms, and tyrosine excites. They compete to enter the brain via the
same route; thus, if there is too much of one or the other, one of them
might lose out.

Neurotransmitters are powerful players in brain function. Scientists
are looking at how various neurotransmitters affect appetite, weight
management, mental illness, and diseases like Parkinson's and amyotrophic lateral sclerosis (Lou Gehrig's disease).

We need to eat protein daily to maintain the supply of amino acids
to the brain. The protein we get from food generally gives us all the
amino acids we need for a healthy brain and body.

☞ Neurotransmitters are the chemicals that transmit messages in the brain.

☞ Neurotransmitters are made up of amino acids we get in our diet.

☞ Amino acids are precursors to neurotransmitters, meaning they are turned into neurotransmitters.

☞ Neurotransmitters are dynamic substances that affect mood, appetite, memory, cognition, arousal, relaxation, muscle performance, and many other aspects of daily life.

☞ Pay attention to your dreams!

## Water into Wine

Let's review a few of the amino acids that are part of a normal diet and are converted into neurotransmitters in the brain. Amino acids that are transformed into neurotransmitters in the brain are called precursors. A precursor is a substance from which another substance is created. If you could turn water into wine, then water would be considered a precursor to wine. Alas, science has not figured that one out yet.

### Tryptophan

Tryptophan is an amino acid found in foods such as chicken, beans, and fish. Tryptophan is a precursor to the neurotransmitter serotonin. Once we eat a food that contains tryptophan, it is then turned into serotonin via a series of chemical steps. Serotonin has been linked with appetite, weight loss, mood, aggression, sleep patterns, and social behaviors, among other things. Prozac and other antidepressant medications all directly affect levels of serotonin in the brain on a pharmacological level (at the amounts found in prescription medications, not in supplements or food). Serotonin is thought of as a "calming" neurotransmitter.

*Mood Rings.* Eating one particular food will not necessarily change your mood or depress your appetite. Since tryptophan is used to make serotonin and serotonin is a calming neurotransmitter, you might think that a meal high in tryptophan could calm you down. But that is not the case. Other amino acids, such as phenylalanine, leucine, and methionine, all take the same train to the Brain Central Station. Therefore the entry of tryptophan into the brain is related to how much tryptophan is in the blood and how much there is in relation to all the other amino acids. Just because an amino acid like tryptophan is in the bloodstream does not necessarily mean it can get into the brain.

---

Serotonin, a neurotransmitter, is made from the amino acid tryptophan, which we get from food. It is linked to mood, appetite, and aggression, among other things. How much serotonin is in the brain depends on many factors, including what you eat.

---

*Thanksgiving Myths.* It is widely believed that the reason everyone turns into slugs after the Thanksgiving meal is that the tryptophan in the turkey makes you sleepy. Tryptophan is necessary for the production of serotonin in the brain, and serotonin is a calming neurotransmitter. However, there are a whole lot of other amino acids, carbohydrates, and fats in that big meal that are jockeying for entry into the brain. The real reasons everyone is glued to the couch after the Thanksgiving meal are overeating, overdrinking, and listening to Uncle John recount the details of his colonoscopy for the 78th time.

### Tyrosine and Phenylalanine

Tyrosine is an indispensable amino acid because it is the precursor to a group of neurotransmitters called catecholamines. The catecholamines are dopamine, norepinephrine, and epinephrine. Catecholamines are associated with numerous brain functions, blood pressure, muscle performance, and mood. They are regarded as excitatory neurotransmitters because they tend to rev up the body and the brain.

Phenylalanine, another important amino acid, is linked to tyrosine because it is a precursor to tyrosine. You can get tyrosine in your diet through foods that contain tyrosine or phenylalanine:

Soy beans
Tofu
Poultry
Fish
Low-fat and nonfat milk, yogurt, and cheese
Lima beans
Pumpkin seeds
Almonds
Bananas

Tyrosine is an amino acid that we get through our diet. It is a precursor to a group of amino acids called catecholamines. Phenylalanine also comes from protein we eat and can be turned into tyrosine in the body.

---

### Save Your Dough

*There are hundreds of Internet sites promoting the sale of over-the-counter amino acid supplements claiming they can do everything from ultra enhancing sports performance to easy weight loss to curing depression. There is no solid scientific evidence to support any of these claims, so don't waste your money.*

---

### Catecholamines

The neurotransmitters epinephrine and norepinephrine (also known as adrenaline and noradrenaline) are catecholamines. Imagine you are in the mall and suddenly here is an announcement over the PA that the "Genuine Stuff" shop is having a huge sale. All Prada bags are 75 percent off, and the latest Caldwell golf clubs are 50 percent off. Imagine the mad dash you and everyone else make for the store. You heart is racing, eyes dilated, breathing heavily, as you race to grab your dream putter before anyone else. Your body has launched into the fight-or-flight mode ignited by the release of catecholamines. When your stress level skyrockets, your body responds. Fight or flight is a survival response in the body, and epinephrine and norepinephrine are key players. All the physiological effects, such as heart pounding and big eyes (for a better field of vision), prepare you to either fight for your life or run for it.

Your body does not differentiate between a life-threatening situation or a money-saving opportunity. If you mentally perceive a situation as a stressor, your body flips on the stress response. Occasional bouts of acute stress do not have unhealthy physiological consequences. Chronic stress does. This brings up a few key points about brain health. The first is that chronic stress that comes from struggles at work, in traffic, and with family can wear out your body and its defense systems. The second is that when you get stressed your body does not know whether you have to fight for your life or you just had a fight with your spouse. The third is that if the stress is chronic, then the flight-or-fight response is in overdrive, which can create some serious health problems. Research suggests that chronic stress can precipitate depression, poor memory, and diseases such as cardiovascular disease and can affect brain function. Managing stress can help keep brain chemicals in balance and your body healthy.

---

No matter what the source of stress is, your body will respond as if it is in a life-threatening situation. Chronic stress wreaks havoc in the body and increases the risk of disease and cognitive decline and may cause atrophy in certain regions of the brain. So unless you want your brain to disintegrate, chill out.

---

*Managing Stress.* "I can't *manage* stress," sneered one of my cardiac patients. "Life is stressful. You can't just make stress go away." When he walked into my office, he took out two PDAs, two cell phones, and a beeper and put them on the desk and said, "Look I have some important calls coming in so I will have to take them." He was a little peeved when I suggested his stress level needed to be addressed.

Managing stress does not mean ignoring it or pretending it does not exist. Life is stressful and seems to be getting more so every day. But there are ways to help your mind and body deal with stress so that it does not eventually strip your gears. Simple steps like taking deep breaths can help. Keeping things in perspective is a good way to defuse an impending stress response. A psychologist I know tells this story:

> It was my wedding day. We were outside in a garden under the chuppah when it started to rain. The dark clouds roiled above, and the rain quickly became torrential. We all got drenched as we ran inside the reception hall. My new mother-in-law was getting very agitated. "Oh, this is awful. Just horrible." She moaned, verging on a full-blown whining attack. I turned to her and said, "No, Sylvia. This is not awful or horrible. Awful is when your child has cancer. Think of the Holocaust when you think of horrible. This is just a little inconvenient, and we will all have a wonderful time." And we did.

We tend to "awfulize" events in our lives and make them far more stressful than need be. While getting yelled at by your boss or being late for an important appointment can be upsetting, they do not have to send you into a major freak-out. The next time you are in a stressful situation, say, stuck in traffic, take a moment to look at the reality of the circumstances. You can sit there and be annoyed and stressed, which won't make the cars move any faster, or you can take a few deep breaths, get an attitude adjustment, turn on some music, and rock out.

*Stress—It Starts in Your Head and Goes to Your Mouth and Your Waistline.* Betty is a young woman with three little children and works part-time. She started coming for nutrition counseling because she said she was desperate to lose weight and get healthy. One day she came in to my office upset. "I am finding it hard to remember to eat well and make healthy choices. I am constantly going back to my comfort foods like cheese and chocolate." She was stressed out and understandably tired. Her stress levels and fatigue were affecting her memory and her coping skills, and she was stress-eating.

For many people stress can trigger emotional eating. In fact, research suggests that one of the reasons people eat when they are stressed is a survival response to the stress hormones in the body. Epinephrine, norepinephrine, and cortisol are poured into the bloodstream when you get stressed. Cortisol levels increase during chronic stress and influence eating behaviors. Scientists have found that when people are chronically stressed they tend to eat high-fat, high-sugar foods that can ultimately lead to weight gain. A study published in the journal *Health Psychology* showed that the stress of daily hassles caused the 422 participants to eat high-fat and high-sugar snacks and eat fewer main meals and vegetables.

Chronic stress can influence your food choices. It's awfully hard to go for the hummus and carrots when your body is telling you it needs M&Ms.

## What to Do

Learning strategies to deal with stressful times is helpful. It is not in the scope of this book to delve into the realm of stress-management techniques, but here are a few simple things you can do.

- Take three to five slow, deep breaths, which helps shut off the flight-or-fight response.
- Take time to understand what your stressors are.
- Make a list of things to do when you are stressed that do not include eating—e.g., taking a walk, listening to music, playing with the dog, creating a new game with your kids, doing laundry.
- Stock your pantry with healthy foods and dump the junk. This way even if you are in a stressful funk, you will only have healthy food to grab.

Catecholamines are initiators of the body's stress response. Chronic stress can increase the risk of disease and have a bad effect on brain function and structure. Learning stress management techniques will help your body stay healthy and your brain stay sharp.

*Dopamine.* Dopamine is another catecholamine whose precursor is the amino acid tyrosine. Dopamine is involved with motor (muscle) function, moods, arousal, learning, pleasure, and reward. In fact, some experts believe that eating highly palatable foods (foods high in sugar, fat, and salt) increases dopamine levels in the brain, so we associate these foods with reward and pleasure. That is why when a delicious food is within our grasp we dive for it knowing it will make us feel good. This is one reason, scientists speculate, that trying to resist our favorite high-calorie foods is so difficult.

Karen was so pleased with herself. She had been to an outdoor barbeque birthday party. "I had salad and grilled chicken," she gushed. "I didn't even want the hot dogs or potato salad. And I did not even eat any birthday cake. It was marvelous." "Good for you, Karen. That is a big step in the right direction," I praised her. She paused and added, "I was so happy that I had been disciplined at the party that when I got home I rewarded myself with a bowl of ice cream." Sometimes we need to retrain our brain and redefine the meaning of "reward."

Dopamine is also implicated in Parkinson's disease as well as age-related cognitive decline and some forms of dementia. These problems arise when the brain either cannot make enough dopamine or cannot use what is available.

## Choline

Although choline, which is considered an essential nutrient, is not an amino acid, it is included here because it is a precursor to the neurotransmitter acetylcholine. We get choline from the food we eat; however, it is not present in a lot of foods. We usually eat it in the form of lecithin. Lecithin is a type of fat that contains choline and is easier to find in food. Lecithin is found in foods such as soybeans, wheat germ, egg yolks, cauliflower, and peanuts. When you eat lecithin, the choline

**Choline Fact:** Human breast milk contains choline to help the baby's brain develop properly.

is teased out of the molecule during digestion and used by the body for various functions. Choline is necessary for a healthy liver, for cell function, and for making acetylcholine.

---

Choline is an essential nutrient. The body needs it to make the neurotransmitter acetylcholine. Choline is also an important substance in brain development in growing fetuses and neonates (infants). It may be important in maintaining or boosting memory, but since most of the scientific studies looking at supplemental choline (taking it as a pill) have been done in rats, we really do not know about the effects of choline supplementation on memory in humans. We get choline from food, usually in the form of lecithin.

---

### Acetylcholine

Acetylcholine is a very active neurotransmitter in the brain and throughout the body. In the brain acetylcholine is linked to arousal, learning, and memory. Scientists suspect that as we age our brain is less able to use actelycholine, and this may have an effect on cognitive decline and the development of Alzheimer's disease.

---

Eating healthy protein every day supplies the brain with the ingredients it needs to make neurotransmitters. Neurotransmitters such as serotonin, dopamine and other catecholamines, and acetylcholine are like members of a dance company performing the complicated and intricate choreography of communication in the brain.

---

☞    Tryptophan is a precursor to serotonin.

☞    Tyrosine is a precursor to the catecholamines.

☞    Phenylalanine is a precursor to tyrosine.

☞   Choline is a precursor to acetylcholine.

☞   Catecholamines can help you get the Prada bag you've always wanted!

## Neurotransmitters and Depression

*Scientists believe that depression results from neurochemical imbalances in the brain. Meaning, the brain chemicals are out of whack. There are too much of some and not enough of others. Deficiencies of serotonin or norephinephrine have both been implicated in clinical depression. Antidepressant medications manipulate brain chemistry to increase levels of serotonin and norepinephrine and have also been used to help people control their weight. Can diet make a difference in depression and obesity? Does eating or craving carbohydrates change someone's mood? There are many theories and studies examining depression, obesity, carbohydrate cravings, and food intake, but for now nothing conclusive can be said. The effects of food on mood are difficult to quantify, since human physiology, biochemistry, and psychology are all intertwined and very variable.*

## Protein and the Rest of You

Healthy Benefits of Protein beyond the Brain

- Healthy protein may help with weight loss.
- Diets high in vegetables and vegetable protein may help lower blood pressure.
- Reducing refined carbohydrates and replacing them with healthy protein may lower the risk of cardiovascular disease and improve cholesterol numbers.
- Cutting down on "bad" carbs (see the carbohydrate chapter for more info) and replacing them with healthy protein may help reduce your waistline.

How much protein do we need? For most of us the recommendation for protein is 0.8 gram per kg of body weight daily. For a 125-pound woman, that would mean about 45 grams of protein a day. A cup of fat-free plain yogurt with berries for breakfast, PB&J for lunch, and 3 ounces of fish for dinner, and you've met your daily protein requirement. For a 185-pound man, that would add up to about 67 grams of protein a day.

People who exercise regularly may need to increase their dietary protein to between 1.2 and 1.4 grams per kg of body weight a day. For people who lift weights, between 1.6 and 1.8 grams per kg per day is recommended. Pregnant and breast-feeding women should get about 71 grams of protein a day. The consensus is that even if you exercise regularly and/or strength-train, you can get all the protein you need through your diet rather than supplements. Even the muscle heads in the gym do not need all the protein-amino shakes and pills they are so fond of if they are eating a healthy diet.

## Plant Proteins

Most folks know that protein comes from animal foods. Few are aware that there are many plant foods that offer excellent sources of protein, too.

**Protein in Selected Foods**

| Food | Amount | Grams |
|---|---|---|
| Halibut, broiled | 3 oz | 15.66 |
| Almonds, dry roasted | 12 | 3.13 |
| Fat-free milk | 8 oz | 8.26 |
| Egg white | 1 | 3.6 |
| Peanut butter | 2 tbs | 9.0 |
| Fat-free plain yogurt | 8 oz | 20.0 |
| Edamame (soy beans) | ½ cup | 8.4 |
| Extrafirm tofu | 3.5 oz | 10.1 |
| Whole-wheat bread | 1 slice | 3.6 |
| Brown rice, cooked | ½ cup | 2.5 |

*Source:* Adapted from USDA National Nutrient Database for Standard Reference, Release 20, United States Department of Agriculture, Agricultural Research Service, 2007, www.ars.usda.gov/ba/bhnrc/ndl.

> *To translate pounds into kilograms, divide by 2.2. For example: 125*
> *pounds / 2.2 = 56.8 kg. To estimate your protein requirements,*
> *multiply your weight in kilograms by the protein recommendations. A*
> *56.8-kg woman would need about 45 grams of protein a day. If she*
> *exercises regularly, she may need 70–80 grams of protein a day.*

## Toot Toot

Who can forget the bean-eating, cowboy tooting scene around the campfire in the movie *Blazing Saddles*? It launched a whole beanophobic culture. While the "toot factor" remains an issue for some people, the health benefits of beans clearly outweigh the fear of tooting. Generally beans, also known as legumes, are considered carbohydrates, but they are also a good source of plant protein. Beans include chick peas, black-eyed peas, lentils, and black, pinto, cannellini, and kidney beans. Buying the dry beans and soaking them overnight is swell. If you do not have the time to do that, canned beans are convenient and affordable.

Beans have big molecules that are not always fully digested. When these big molecules get to the large intestine, they provide a nice meal for the healthy bacteria that live in the colon. It is the bacteria in the colon that produce tooting gas. For many people, the body adapts to regular bean consumption, so there is less gas. If you have a gas problem when you eat beans, try an over-the-counter product like Beano. Eating beans in a pureed form like a dip or hummus may help reduce gas too.

Beans are high in antioxidants, vitamins, minerals, and fiber. They are not naturally high in sodium, but sodium is added to the packing water of canned beans. Rinsing the canned beans in a sieve before using will help remove some of the added sodium. Organic canned beans have less sodium added. A few popular brands of canned beans are now offering "low sodium" and organic options. Beans you may not have heard of but are worth a try: mung, adzuki.

## What Beans Can Do for You

- Including beans in your diet several times a week may decrease the risk of colorectal adenomas (polyps), which may in turn lower the risk of colorectal cancer.
- Eating beans regularly may lower the risk of coronary heart disease.
- The Shanghai Women's Health Study looked at the legume consumption of more than 64,000 women and their risk of developing type 2 diabetes. Researchers found that consumption of legumes, particularly soybeans, was inversely associated with the risk of type 2 diabetes. The more legumes these women ate, the lower their risk of getting type 2 diabetes.
- Beans are hearty and are a good alternative to high-fat protein sources like red meat.
- In the Nurses' Health Study of 83,818 women, researchers found that women who ate peanuts and peanut butter had a lower risk of type 2 diabetes. Peanuts, which technically are considered a legume, are high in healthy fats, magnesium, and fiber.
- If you have not seen *Blazing Saddles*, rent the DVD. It will fill your brain's daily quota for good satiric humor (and your kids will think you're really cool, too).

## What You Can Do with Beans

- Make hummus
- Make a white bean dip
- Add to soups and stews
- Add to pasta
- Serve as a side dish
- Use dried beans to create fun art and decorative projects (creativity is good for the brain, too).

## Full of (Soy)Beans

Soybeans, also known as edamame, can be used in a variety of forms, including soy milk, soy sauce, yuba, tofu, miso, tempeh, and soy nuts. Soybeans are thought to have been domesticated in China as early as the eleventh century BC, but history is sketchy, since Google wasn't around then. Eventually the soybean made it to the United States.

According to soy experts, Samuel Bowen, a former seaman employed by the East India Company, brought soybeans to Savannah, the colony of Georgia, from China via London in 1765. In 1770 Benjamin Franklin sent soybean seeds from England to his botanist friend John Bartram in Philadelphia. Thus a seed for what has become one of the United States' biggest crops was planted. In 2007 the United States exported 1 billion bushels of soybeans, which accounted for 37 percent of the world's soybean trade. That's a lot of beans. Soy is an excellent source of plant protein because it contains all the essential amino acids adults need. Approximately 40 percent of the calories in soy come from protein. Soy contains omega-3 fats, B vitamins, and phytoestrogens. Phytoestrogens are plant compounds that are similar to, but weaker than, the human hormone estrogen. The phytoestrogens in soy are called isoflavones, and these compounds are thought to provide some of soy's health benefits.

---

Soy originally came from China a really long time ago. Soybeans are used for food, oils, and even biodiesel fuel. Soy contains lots of healthy stuff like protein, vitamins, omega-3 fats, antioxidants, and isoflavones.

---

### To Fu or Not to Fu

Tofu is a curd made from the soybean and has been used as a source of dietary protein for centuries. The invention of tofu in China dates from as early as AD 200–900. Tofu moved from China to Korea, Japan, Indonesia, Thailand, and Nepal to become a staple in Asian cuisines. Tofu is a versatile food and comes in several consistencies, including silken, firm, and extra firm. I use the silken to make creamy sauces and soups and the extra firm in stir fries and pasta sauces.

Americans are eating more tofu than ever before, yet it remains a misunderstood food. I made baked marinated tofu for a party I was having. When I offered some to my friend James, he pursed his lips shut, crinkled his brow, and ducked, as if I was trying to give him bad-tasting cough medicine. "Ugh! I hate tofu," he grimaced. Force-feeding party guests is a serious breach of good manners, so I gave in gracefully. I'll

### Soy of Many Faces

*Edamame:* The green soybean. You can buy them frozen (do not eat the pods) and use them as a side dish, in soups or sauces, or to make dips.

*Tofu:* A curd made from soybeans.

*Yuba:* Soy milk skin. When soy milk is heated, a thin, protein rich skin forms on the top. The skin, called yuba, is sold fresh or dried and is used in Asian cuisines.

*Soy milk:* Made from soaked soybeans that have been finely ground and strained.

*Miso:* Soybeans fermented with rice, salt, and a mild culture and then aged. Used frequently in Japanese cuisine.

*Tempeh:* Soybeans sometimes mixed with grains such as rice and fermented into a cake. Imparts a smoky flavor. Traditional in Indonesian foods.

*Soy nuts:* Soybeans that have been soaked in water and then roasted.

*Soy sauce:* The common high-sodium, dark brown liquid made from fermenting soybeans.

tell you a secret. James loved the tofu vegetable lasagna I served at a Christmas party a few months later. I did not tell him it was made with tofu.

Tofu is a healthy, versatile food. Don't be afraid to experiment with it in different dishes. Do not attempt to force-feed tofu to your guests.

There has been some controversy associated with tofu lately. A few studies have found that middle-aged and older people who consumed tofu regularly showed signs of decreased cognitive function. These studies

## Don't Believe Everything You Read

*There is a lot of really bad, downright stupid information on the Internet. It is written in such a way that it all sounds very plausible and very true. While doing research for this chapter, I came across an Internet article on a right-wing, ultraconservative Web site that says it is undeniable that eating soy is "making our kids gay." The article says that soy is "a slow poison that's severely damaging our children and threatening to tear apart our culture." There are so many reasons this is silly and paranoid that it is not worth discussing, except as an example of ridiculous rants that saturate the Internet. If you need information, go to reputable sites. Sites with .edu, .gov, or .org are good places to start, though not a guarantee of accurate information.*

have been a cause for concern. They have several limitations, including methodological and statistical issues. It is important to note that these are preliminary findings, and there are many studies that highlight the potential health benefits of eating soy foods, including protection from cardiovascular disease, some cancers, high blood pressure, stroke, heart attack, and cognitive decline. Due to soy's high content of polyunsaturated (healthy) fats, fiber, vitamins, and minerals and low content of saturated fat, the American Heart Association recommends including soy as part of a heart healthy diet. More research needs to be done to determine whether eating soy or tofu has an effect on cognitive decline. Soy may have a detrimental effect only if consumed after a certain age and in a certain quantity. In the meantime, experts are recommending that we consume soy foods such as tofu, tempeh, and edamame as part of a healthful diet and that we avoid taking soy supplements.

A few scientific studies have suggested that tofu (not soybeans) may be related to cognitive decline. The studies had limitations, so we really don't know whether we can link tofu to cognitive decline.

☞ Unlike Google, soybeans have been around for centuries.

☞ Soy is a good source of plant protein.

☞ Tofu, a curd made from soy, is a versatile food that has been used in the Far East for centuries.

☞ Tofu may have positive or negative effects on the brain.

☞ James likes tofu!

### Tofu and Cognitive Function—The Study Everyone Is Talking About

A study published in the journal *Dementia and Geriatric Cognitive Disorders* in the spring of 2008 carried the title "High Tofu Intake Is Associated with Worse Memory in Elderly Indonesian Men and Women." The study found that tempeh, a fermented form of soy curd, seems to protect memory, while tofu, which is not fermented, was associated with worse memory. The scientists were not sure why they got these results. One factor that could potentially have a significant impact on the study findings is that tofu is processed with formaldehyde, which is used as a preservative in Indonesia. The U.S. Embassy reports that fresh noodles, preserved fish, and tofu contain high levels of formaldehyde, a chemical used in embalming fluid. Tempeh does not. The *Jakarta Post* (February 28, 2008) quoted lead study author Professor Eef Hogervorst as saying, "The culprit [for memory loss associated with tofu consumption] may be formaldehyde but we need further study to confirm this."

Scientists pondered other reasons for the results, including how phytoestrogens in soy, a plant chemical that is similar to the human hormone estrogen, might affect memory in people over 65. Tempeh, they speculate, is high in the B vitamin folate. Folate has protective effects on brain function and is associated with lower dementia risk.

A scientific study found that in Indonesia high tofu consumption was associated with worsening memory function, especially in people over the age of 68. Scientists do not know whether this might be due to the phytoestrogens or potential toxins like formaldehyde, which is commonly found in tofu processed in Indonesia.

## Soup to Nuts

"I cannot seem to lose any weight," complained a patient of mine. "I am eating healthier than ever. I stopped the roast beef sandwiches and cheese. What's going on?"

I probed further into what he was eating. It turns out he took my advice and began snacking on nuts instead of sweets and junk food. The problem was he was eating up to 2 pounds of nuts every day. No wonder he was not losing weight. The health benefits of nuts are well documented. They are cardio-protective and may help lower the risk of diabetes, metabolic syndrome, coronary heart disease, and colon cancer in women, and they may reduce inflammation. Nuts and seeds are a good source of plant protein and contain healthy fats, fiber, vitamins, minerals and antioxidants. They do not, as many people believe, contain any cholesterol. Nuts are high in calories, so you need to watch how much you are eating. A handful of nuts is about 100 calories. All nuts are good, so buy them unsalted and opt for a variety. Nut butters are good too: peanut, almond, and cashew butters are delicious (2 tablespoons = 190 calories). A favorite hiking sandwich of mine is peanut butter and banana. Get the "natural" kind of nut butters with no added salt or sugar.

All nuts provide health benefits including protein, vitamins, minerals, and unsaturated fats. They are good for your heart and brain. But they are high in calories, so watch how much you eat.

☞   Nuts are a good source of plant protein.

☞   Nuts contain healthy fats and fiber.

☞   Nuts offer many health benefits.

## Walnuts

Walnuts are a good source of healthy omega-3 fats and protein. Eating walnuts is good for the heart, may help reduce the risk of diabetes, lower blood pressure and cholesterol, and may reduce inflammation. Cardiovascular disease, high blood pressure, and diabetes are risk factors for dementia. About an ounce of walnuts (⅓ cup) contains 185 calories, 4 grams of protein, and 2.6 grams of omega-3 fats. A small study found that as few as four walnuts a day increased omega-3 fats in the body. Walnuts are a great afternoon snack with a cup of tea, fat-free milk, or flavored seltzer. Use walnuts in cereal, salads, pastas, soups, and smoothies.

## Brazil Nuts

Plant foods like Brazil nuts are the major dietary sources of selenium. Selenium is a trace mineral that works with other compounds as a powerful antioxidant. It may help protect brain cells from oxidative damage. Research is suggesting that there is an increased risk of cognitive decline with declining levels of selenium. Just one or two Brazil nuts a day, or a few times a week, can up your selenium levels. But don't overdo it. Our bodies can handle only a tiny amount of selenium at a time.

## Almonds

Almonds, high in vitamin E, help reduce LDL (bad cholesterol) oxidation, which means almonds help stop gunk from building up in your arteries. Almonds also have strong antioxidant properties that come from health-promoting plant compounds called flavonoids.

## Cashews

There is not a lot of research on cashews and their effects on health, but they are included in the general "nut" category in the medical literature that says nuts are healthy. Cashews contain important minerals such as copper and magnesium. My friend Tom loves to use chopped cashews as a topping for vegetarian chili.

**Going Nuts**

| Nut or Seed | Amount | Calories | Fat grams | Protein grams |
|---|---|---|---|---|
| Walnuts | 1 oz | 185 | 19 | 4.3 |
| Brazil Nuts | 4 nuts | 131 | 13.2 | 3 |
| Almonds | 1 oz | 169 | 15 | 6 |
| Cashews | 1 oz | 163 | 13 | 4 |
| Flaxseeds, ground | 1 tbs | 37 | 3 | 1.3 |
| Pumpkin | 1 oz | 148 | 12 | 9.4 |
| Sunflower Seeds | 1 oz | 164 | 14.4 | 6 |
| Sesame Seeds | 1 tbs | 50 | 5 | 2 |

Source: Adapted from USDA National Nutrient Database for Standard Reference, Release 20, United States Department of Agriculture, Agricultural Research Service, 2007, www.ars.usda.gov/ba/bhnrc/ndl.

## The Good Seed

Seeds like flax, pumpkin, sunflower, and sesame offer a lot more than a little protein. They are high in vitamins, minerals, healthy fats, and phytochemicals. Flaxseeds are high in omega-3 fats. Pumpkin seeds are high in manganese and magnesium. Sunflower seeds are a good source of vitamin E and thiamin. And sesame seeds contain copper, tryptophan, and calcium. Add to salads, yogurt, cereals, or muffins.

## The Good, the Bad, and the Debate

Most proteins in animal foods have all the amino acids your body needs, meaning they are "complete" proteins. Plant proteins tend to be incomplete, meaning not all the amino acids your body needs are in a single food. Back in the 1970s there was the notion that vegetarians had to eat protein foods in combination with one another to get a balance of amino acids. Like brown rice and beans. We have since learned that this is not the case. Vegetarians or people lowering their intake of animal foods can eat a variety of healthy protein throughout the day to achieve a balanced intake of amino acids.

The problem with animal protein is that it is usually tied up with bad saturated fat and is high in calories. In addition, research is finding that diets high in red meat and/or processed meats may increase the risk of type 2 diabetes, colorectal cancer, mortality, coronary heart disease, breast cancer, esophageal, liver, and lung cancers, and chronic obstructive lung disease.

I am one of the few dietitians who will tell you that there are bad foods in this world and red and processed meats are two of them. That does not mean you cannot have red meat on rare occasions. It is when you eat red or processed meats regularly, every day or several times a week, that problems arise. "But we are born carnivores," objected one of my patients. People can get quite steamed when they are told meat is bad for them or even think someone might say that. I was on a television set one morning to do a nutrition segment on healing foods like turmeric, ginger, and berries. The producer was showing me how she had arranged the props when the news anchor with whom I was to do the segment came on the set. The producer introduced me, and I said, "Hello. It is nice to meet you." The news anchor glared at me and said

### Tiring of Matilda

*Peri- and postmenopausal women have a tough time losing weight. It's just not fair. My friend Laurie actually named the tire around her middle. "I'd like to introduce you," she says as she pinches her waistline roll of fat, "to Matilda." No matter how tenacious Matilda is at sticking around, it is always a good idea to exercise and to eat healthy foods. If you are trying to lose weight, be careful what foods you choose to limit. A study in the* Journal of the American Dietetic Association *found that postmenopausal women who were trying to lose weight and were not eating enough protein lost muscle mass. It is better to cut down on carbohydrates like bread, cookies, or rice and keep the healthy protein in your daily diet.*

defensively, "I am a carnivore, and I have no intention of changing." I looked back and said, "OK." He had not even said "Hullo."

The truth is that even if we are born carnivores, our bodies were not meant to withstand the titanic amount of saturated fat, meat, and processed meats people eat today. Your body does not know there are grocery stores, pizza delivery, or restaurants. Your body thinks you have to go out and catch breakfast every day. The human body is designed to handle only small amounts of saturated fat over time. The average consumption of meat in the United States in 2002 was 200 pounds per person, 23 pounds higher than in 1970. A 6-ounce piece of broiled filet mignon has 541 calories and 40 grams of fat, 16 grams of them saturated. That is almost a whole day's worth of bad fat. In one year, eating 200 pounds of steak (I am using one type of meat for simplicity) would mean you ate 8,690 grams of saturated fat, just from meat. That does not include cheese, ice cream, butter, or other high-fat animal foods. We are not even addressing the chemicals that are added to and that form in processed, cured, or smoked meats. Science and biochemistry tell us that saturated fat and red and processed meats increase inflammation, which leads to diseases such as dementia and heart disease. Assaulting your body with upwards of 20 pounds of saturated fat a year just isn't a good thing.

Libby is an overweight woman in her sixties. She and her husband love meat. She said they eat it every day. She also loves cheese. Libby's doctor told her that if she keeps going the way she's going, she will become a type 2 diabetic. It was just a matter of time. When I suggested she drastically lower her meat and cheese consumption, she looked at me as if I had asked her to shave her head. "There is no way we could give up meat. My husband wouldn't hear of it." She and I talked this over, and she agreed to try to limit red meat to once a week. Several weeks later Libby came in and admitted, "You know we only have meat once, sometimes twice a week, and I don't miss it at all. I've really cut down on the cheese, too." She paused. "I tried a veggie burger. It was so good. Now when my husband grills his meat, I can have my veggie burger." Libby is like a lot of people who feel that limiting meat, butter, cheese, and other proteins and fats from animals would be nearly impossible. In my practice, very few people, upon seriously reducing their animal food consumption, tell me they miss it. More often than not people tell me they do not miss it and feel better than they ever thought they could. They have also adopted other healthy lifestyle changes, such as eating more fruits, vegetables, and whole grains and exercising. When you feel better, your mood improves and your brain function ratchets up several notches. If you choose to eat animal protein, stick with the leanest possible cuts and keep portion sizes to 3–4 ounces a serving. White-meat poultry (no skin), nonfat dairy foods like cheese and yogurt, fish, and eggs are your best bets. Keep the roast beef, brie, and burgers for rare occasions.

---

Animal protein is usually tied up with bad saturated fat. In addition, red and processed meats increase the risk of chronic diseases. You are better off restricting your consumption of red and processed meats to rare occasions. It's better for your health, the environment, and the animals.

---

☞   Most animal protein has all the essential amino acids your body needs.

☞   Plant proteins have many essential amino acids but not usually all in one food.

☞   Combining plant proteins to create a "complete" protein is a thing of the past.

☞   Eating high-fat animal foods and red and processed meats is bad for you.

☞   There are good and bad foods.

☞   You can eat bad foods on rare occasions.

## Brain-Boosting Breakfast Ideas

The first three items in this list are available at many delis and diners.

- Egg-white (or egg-substitute) omelet with spinach, onions, peppers (any vegetable is fine here). Cook in a small bit of olive oil or in a nonstick pan. Serve with a slice of whole-grain bread with a schmeer of vegan margarine.
- PB&J on a whole-wheat English muffin
- Low-fat cottage cheese with ¼ slice of melon
- Whole-grain cereal (cold or hot) with fat-free milk + 2 teaspoons of toasted wheat germ, ½ cup berries, or ½ banana
- Whole-wheat tortilla stuffed with scrambled egg substitute topped with salsa
- One to two slices of whole-grain toast with melted low-fat cheese and tomato slices
- Leftover healthy pizza (no cheese or part-skim mozzarella) and lots of vegetables
- Hearty multi-whole-grain bread French toast topped with a dab of maple syrup and a sprinkling of pumpkin seeds (about 1 teaspoon)
- Beverages: fat-free milk, coffee, tea, 4–6 ounces of 100 percent juice, water, seltzer, juice spritzer (3 ounces juice mixed with 5 ounces of seltzer)

## The Best Healthy Protein

Buy organic whenever possible.

Organic egg whites
Soy—edamame, tofu, tempeh
Nuts—all are good—unsalted
Beans/legumes
Low-fat and nonfat dairy foods like fat-free milk and yogurt
Fish (but see Chapter 1)

- Protein is made up of amino acids.
- Amino acids are the main ingredients for neurotransmitters.
- Neurotransmitters are what the brain uses to communicate among its zillions of neurons.
- Neurotransmitters are powerful chemicals that affect mood, appetite, arousal, energy, and much more.
- Your brain needs a constant supply of amino acids every day.
- Healthy protein comes from both plants and animals.
- Animal protein is usually tied up with bad saturated fat.
- Low-fat animal protein includes nonfat dairy foods, white-meat poultry, fish, and eggs.
- Plant proteins include nuts, seeds, soy, beans, and grains.

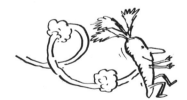

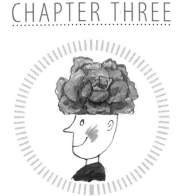

## CHAPTER THREE

# The Sugar Brain Express: Carbohydrates

───── KEY POINTS ─────

⇨ The brain uses a lot of energy.

⇨ Glucose is the primary and preferred source of fuel for the brain.

⇨ Glucose has to come from food known as carbohydrates.

⇨ Carbohydrates come in many forms including bread, vegetables, fruits, and beans.

⇨ The brain needs a constant supply of glucose to function properly.

⇨ **Carbohydrates get broken down into glucose and carried to all the cells in the body for fuel.**

⇨ **Insulin escorts glucose out of the blood vessels into the cells.**

⇨ **There are good carbohydrates and junky carbohydrates.**

⇨ **Fruits and vegetables are really, really good for your brain.**

—— NUTRITION PRESCRIPTION ——
*for* CARBOHYDRATES

⇨ **Choose whole grains like whole-wheat bread, whole-grain cereals, whole-grain pastas, muffins, and waffles.**

⇨ **Eat tons of vegetables every day.**

⇨ **Have a few pieces of fruit every day.**

### The Utility Bill

EVEN THOUGH THE HUMAN brain accounts for only 2 percent of the weight of the whole body, it uses a good 20 percent of the body's total energy. The brain uses more energy than any organ in the body. You'd break the bank if you had to pay that electric bill. My electric company, which I called recently to find out how to lower my bill, told me that anything with a motor (like my dehumidifier) hikes energy costs. My solution to lowering the energy bill was to use only one of my two basement dehumidifiers (hoping one is enough to combat mold and mildew), but you do not want to reduce your brain's energy consumption and nor do you want to skimp on fuel. Your brain is motoring 24/7, and it needs a constant supply of fuel to do so. Even when you are sleeping, your brain is still chugging away, keeping you breathing and dreaming, your heart pumping, and blood flowing. The high-test, affordable, environmentally friendly fuel your brain uses is glucose.

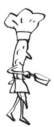

The brain is an energy hog. It uses glucose as its primary, preferred source of fuel. Glucose is also used by the body as a basis for forming neurotransmitters, such as acetylcholine and glutamate, the brain's communication chemicals.

## White Trash

Glucose, also known as blood sugar, comes from carbohydrates. Carbohydrates are critical for a well-functioning brain and for powering muscles. We have to eat carbohydrates to enjoy their energy-boosting benefits. Most people think of starchy foods like potatoes, bread, and pasta when they think of carbohydrates. Carbohydrates also come from fruits, vegetables, beans, grains, milk, and nuts. Carbohydrates contain fiber, vitamins, minerals, healthy fats, antioxidants, and health-promoting compounds called phytochemicals. For the most part, when carbohydrates are taken to their simplest form, they become glucose or fructose. Glucose is the predominant carbohydrate the brain uses for energy and fuel.

Your brain cannot store glucose, so it needs to be bathed in glucose all day long. Throw in some amino acids and you've got yourself a nourishing brain bath. The brain absorbs glucose as it flows past and uses it for petrol. When you don't eat for a while and feel cranky or light headed, it is because your brain needs fuel. A growling stomach is also your body's way of telling you it needs fuel and it's time to eat.

There are good carbohydrates and junky carbohydrates. Experts from the Harvard School of Public Health believe that the kind of carbohydrate you eat may have as much of an impact on the risk of chronic diseases as the kind of fats you eat. You have probably heard that "white food is bad," referring to white bread, white rice, and the like. When I was discussing this in a nutrition class I was teaching, one of my students piped up in her heavy Bronx accent and said, "White food is white ta-rash." It was apt but not 100 percent true, since there are white foods, like cauliflower, that are good for you. It is the refined carbohydrates that we want to limit.

Carbohydrates supply the fuel your brain and body need. Foods like vegetables, fruits, and whole grains supply the brain and body with substances vital for good health and energy. Eating a diet high in refined carbohydrates may increase your risk of heart disease, diabetes, and cognitive decline.

Good looking, so refined, wouldn't you like to know what's going on in my mind? A refined carbohydrate is one that has been milled and had the fiber, bran, germ, and virtually all the naturally occurring vitamins, minerals, protein, fats, and antioxidants removed. What is left is the starchy part of the grain, such as white rice. Refined grains are then enriched, which means some B vitamins and iron are added back into the flour or grain. But it is never as healthy as the original, whole grain. Without the fiber, protein, and healthy fats, refined grains are rapidly absorbed when we eat them.

☞   Carbohydrates are good for you.

☞   Carbohydrates supply the brain and working muscles with fuel.

☞   Glucose is the form of fuel your body uses.

☞   Whole grains supply fuel, vitamins, minerals, fats, and proteins.

☞   Refined grains are best avoided.

## How Carbohydrates Get into the Bloodstream and Cells

It is a good idea to have a basic understanding of how carbohydrates get into the bloodstream and affect blood sugar levels and insulin release. With this bit of knowledge you can make the connection between why good carbohydrates are good and the junky ones are junky, why diabetes is a risk factor for cognitive decline, and how glucose affects the brain, cognition, and energy levels.

## Potatoes and Pearls

Think of a strand of pearls. Each pearl is a molecule of glucose. When pearls are strung together, they become a necklace. When molecules of glucose are strung together, they become a starch molecule. A single starch molecule may have more than 3,000 glucose units all strung together. In a potato or rice grain there can be as many as 1 million starch molecules in 1 cubic inch of food. When you digest starch, the string of glucose units gets pulled apart and the glucose molecules are separated into single units, like single pearls.

---

Starch molecules are made up of glucose molecules that are strung together like a strand of pearls. When you digest starch (or any carbohydrate), it gets broken down into single molecules of glucose. Now the glucose is ready for transport into the bloodstream and to the cells, where it will be used for energy. Fruits, vegetables, beans, and other carbohydrates also contribute to the body's needs for glucose, but they do not yield the concentration of glucose that starchy foods  do.

---

## Route 66

Your arteries are the highways of your body. Their main function is to transport stuff like oxygen, vitamins, water, fats, amino acids, and glucose from one place to another. At various stations or exits along the way, stuff is unloaded into cells and organs. After you eat some bread, for example, and the carbohydrates are digested into glucose molecules, they are absorbed through the gut wall into the bloodstream. Thus it is normal that the levels of glucose in your bloodstream, known as blood sugar, rise after a meal. When your body detects a rise in blood sugar, it jumps into action to get that sugar out of the arteries and into the cells, where it is used for fuel. If blood sugar levels stay high for long periods of time, the sugar can damage your eyes, kidneys, and arteries.

Arteries are like Route 66 and provide the means whereby nutrients, water, oxygen, and other important things are transported through-out the body. When carbohydrates are broken down into glucose, they are absorbed into the bloodstream. This causes a normal rise in blood sugar levels. Your body then works to get the glucose out of the blood and into the cells, where it is used for fuel. As this process proceeds, blood sugar levels drop as glucose is moved from blood into the cells. When levels of glucose in the blood get to a certain low point, you body rings the dinner bell and tells you it's time to eat again.

☞   When carbohydrates get digested, they become molecules of glucose.

☞   Arteries are the highways of the body. Their job is to transport stuff from one place to another.

☞   Glucose travels in the arteries.

☞   Pearls are appropriate for any occasion!

## Escort Services

Glucose needs an escort. It does not freely flow from the arteries into cells. Glucose's escort is called insulin. Insulin is a hormone that has many functions and is made in the pancreas. After you eat a meal, your body detects that the amount of sugar in your blood has risen. The pancreas responds to rising levels of blood sugar by releasing insulin into the bloodstream. Insulin escorts glucose out of the arteries and into each cell.

Without insulin, glucose cannot get out of the arteries to feed the cells, so it stays in the bloodstream. People with diabetes may not have enough insulin, be resistant to the insulin they do produce, or, in the case of type 1 diabetes, do not produce any insulin. Therefore, in people with diabetes, the amount of glucose in the bloodstream stays high unless they learn to manage their blood sugar levels. Tools for managing blood sugar levels include eating healthy food, weight management, exercise, and when necessary taking medications that help lower blood sugar.

Your body keeps a keen eye on blood sugar levels, since your brain needs a constant supply of glucose to function and your body knows that chronic high blood sugar levels are unhealthy.

---

Insulin is the escort service that glucose uses to get from the bloodstream into the cells. Your body tightly regulates blood sugar levels to be sure the brain and other organs are getting a constant supply of fuel.

---

Your brain, however, does not need insulin to escort the glucose from the bloodstream into the cells. The brain uses its own special transport molecule called, aptly, glucose transporter 1 (GLUT 1). Even so, when general blood sugar levels are low, the glucose available to your brain is low, too.

In summary, we have taken starch, like potatoes or bread, from your mouth to the digestive system, where it is broken down into glucose; the glucose from the digestive system into the bloodstream; and the glucose from the bloodstream, with an assist from insulin, into the cells. When you eat regularly, your brain cells are getting a consistent glucose bath throughout the day that feeds and fuels them—a good reason for not skipping meals and depriving your brain of energy.

☞ Glucose needs an escort to get from the bloodstream into cells.

☞ Insulin is the escort that moves glucose out of the arteries.

☞ Insulin is made in the pancreas and helps keep blood sugar levels normal.

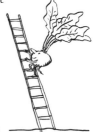

### Tea

*There is nothing like a hot cup of tea to set things right. For centuries tea has been a staple in many cultures. The earliest record of tea and its cultivation comes from China in the fourth century AD. Since then, tea has spanned the globe. Science has done its share of tea promotion by suggesting that both black and green teas have health-promoting benefits. Research suggests that tea is good for the cardiovascular system, reduces internal inflammation, and may be protective against some cancers. Because teas contain antioxidants, there is speculation that drinking tea regularly may also help protect the brain from oxidative stress and cognitive decline. Both black and green teas contain polyphenols, powerful antioxidants, that may be neuroprotective. Instead of an afternoon cup of coffee switch to tea.*

## Junky Carbohydrates

The moment you have been waiting for has arrived. Now the difference between good carbohydrates and junky ones will finally make sense. When you consume foods like white bread, cookies, soda, cakes, pretzels, pastries, and other foods made with white flour or sugar, they get digested quickly. With white flour the reason is that the refining process removes all the fiber, fats, vitamins, minerals, antioxidants, and protein from the original grain and all that is left is the starchy part. White flour is so fine it is like a powder and is rapidly digested and absorbed. Sugar is already in a basic form, so it too gets digested and absorbed into the bloodstream quickly.

Processed carbohydrates like white rice, sweets, and junk food get digested and absorbed into the bloodstream quickly.

## Sodas, Sweetened Drinks: A Cocktail for Obesity, Diabetes, and Brain Drain

*Sugar-sweetened drinks are the largest single source of calories in the U.S. diet. Included are beverages sweetened with sugar or high-fructose corn syrup. People who drink sweetened drinks, including sodas, fruit drinks, and iced teas, regularly, weigh more and are at increased risk of type 2 diabetes. Spend your calories on healthy foods you really enjoy. You can literally save hundreds of calories every day by dumping the soda and sweetened beverages and choosing seltzer, flavored seltzers, water, tea, or coffee instead.*

The quick absorption of carbohydrates causes a dramatic spike in blood sugar levels. Your body responds by dumping insulin into the bloodstream to get blood sugar levels to a normal range. This causes a few problems. In the body when a lot of insulin is poured into the bloodstream, it can accelerate the movement of glucose out of the blood and cause blood sugar levels to drop swiftly. This triggers fatigue and hunger and sometimes crankiness. I call it the sugar wave effect.

"I had such a bad day on Friday," Kelly reported. We looked at her food record, where she had written down everything she had eaten in the past week. For breakfast she had a slice of frozen French toast (toasted, of course) and a diet cola. By midmorning her energy levels tanked, her brain was cobwebbed, and she grabbed the nearest candy from someone's desk. In her food record she wrote "starving" next to the hot dog, hamburger, macaroni salad, potato salad, and dessert she ate at a lunchtime barbeque. "What happened?" she asked. Kelly's day began with an all too common mistake. She had a high-carbohydrate breakfast. She had a piece of white bread coated with sugar, no fiber, and little protein, which started the sugar wave effect. Her blood sugar spiked, then took a nosedive, and by midmorning she was crashing (get the analogy? waves rise up and then crash). She opted for the quick-grab chocolate. By lunch the sugar wave effect had rolled into its second crash of the day, and Kelly was starving.

It is hard to make healthy choices and monitor how much you eat when you are overhungry. The first change Kelly needed to make was to be sure to have whole grains at breakfast with some protein. Whole grains and protein cause a gentler rise in blood sugar followed by an easy decline, so energy levels are not shooting through the roof and falling into the basement in a few short hours. "You are right," Kelly said. "When I have peanut butter and jelly on whole wheat or scrambled egg whites and whole-grain toast in the morning, I never crash and I don't go scavenging for a midmorning snack."

Refined and processed carbohydrates cause a rapid spike followed by a precipitous drop in blood sugar levels, the sugar wave effect. When blood sugar surges, a lot of insulin is dumped into the bloodstream to control the high blood sugar. All that insulin can cause plummeting blood sugar levels that result in fatigue and hunger and ultimately weight gain. More important, over time the cells that make insulin, called beta cells, may burn out because they have been working overtime and have been pushed to their insulin-making limits. To top it off, a diet high in refined carbohydrates increases internal inflammation and is associated with chronic disease.

☞   Junky carbohydrates are absorbed quickly and cause a rapid rise in blood sugar.

☞   Insulin is secreted by the pancreas and is poured into the bloodstream to drop glucose levels.

☞   The drop in blood glucose causes hunger, fatigue, and low blood sugar.

☞   Chronic consumption of junky carbohydrates increases the risk of cognitive decline, diabetes, and other diseases.

---

## The Prestige of Wonder Bread

*Want to be considered royal, rich, and totally cool? Eat white bread.*
*That is, if you are living in Tudor times. Back in Tudor England,*
*between AD 1400 and 1600, white bread was a sign of prestige in*
*high society. White bread was thought of as purer than whole-grain*
*breads. It was more expensive because more refining was necessary. The*
*only people who could afford white bread were the nobility, so it quickly*
*became a status symbol. The nobility dined on very fine white loaves*
*of bread called manchets. The poorer people were sold the hearty, dark,*
*whole-grain breads—hence the name peasant bread.*

---

## Getting High

The glycemic index is a measure of how certain foods we eat affect blood sugar and insulin. Some foods, like white bread and white rice, cause a rapid rise in blood sugar and insulin levels after we eat them, while other foods, such as lentils and carrots, cause a slow increase in glucose and insulin levels. Foods that rank lower on the glycemic index, meaning they cause a slower rise in blood sugar and insulin, are associated with a decreased risk of cardiovascular disease, diabetes. and cognitive decline. People on a low glycemic diet also have better lipid profiles—for example, better cholesterol and triglycerides. The lower-glycemic-index foods have more fiber, protein, and/or fat and thus are digested and absorbed more slowly than refined carbohydrates. Science tells us slower is better. Conversely, people who eat diets high on the glycemic index, including white rice, bread, potatoes, and sodas, are at increased risk of cardiovascular disease and type 2 diabetes.

People are all atwitter about the glycemic index and its cousin the glycemic load. These are confusing terms for most of us. The glycemic load is a mathematical construct of the glycemic index that puts the ranking of foods in a more realistic context. Meaning, it may be a useful research tool, but we don't need to spend time on it. Just know that about 98 percent of your grains should be whole grains. It is a good idea to avoid sweets, white bread, rice, and sodas and other sweetened beverages and concentrate on healthier foods. If you are at an Italian restaurant and whole-wheat pasta isn't available, don't get your panties in a twist. Once in a while refined carbohydrates are perfectly fine.

Good carbohydrates are whole foods like whole-wheat bread, whole-grain pasta, oatmeal, and wild rice as well as fruits, vegetables, beans, and nuts. Junky carbohydrates include white bread and rice, french fries, junk food, and desserts. Making the switch to whole grains is easier than you think. Buy 100 percent whole-grain products. Some of the whole-grain pastas are a blend of white flour and whole wheat, and while a blend is not optimal, it is a step in the right direction. Take a first step and buy whole-wheat English muffins. Then try a whole-grain pasta. Move on to making some brown rice. If you are wedded to white rice, as many cultures are, first try mixing white and brown rices together (cook them separately).

## Whole Grains: Little Miracles

Several studies have shown that eating whole grains decreases the risk of diabetes, metabolic syndrome, stroke, hypertension, inflammation, and heart disease. What more can a girl ask for?

Look for "100 percent whole grains" on the label. In fact, look for the word "*whole.*" Look in the ingredient list. If you see wheat flour, stone ground, organic, seminola or durham wheat, or all natural, it does *not* mean the grains are whole grains. Corn and oats are usually whole. Rolled or steel-cut oats are fine.

## Common Whole Grains

- Brown rice
- Wild rice
- Whole wheat
- Oats and oatmeal
- Pearl barley
- Popcorn
- Whole cornmeal

## Exotic Grains to Try

- Quinoa
- Kasha
- Spelt
- Farro
- Kamut
- Millet
- Amaranth
- Wahini rice
- Black rice (Indonesian black rice)
- Wheat berries

## Whole-Grain Foods

- Whole-wheat pasta
- Whole-grain bread
- Oatmeal
- Oat bran
- Whole-grain cereal
- Shredded wheat
- Corn tortilla
- Whole-wheat wraps
- Buckwheat pancakes
- Rice cakes
- Soy crisps
- Whole-grain pretzels

## Whole Grains a Day—Some Ideas

- Whole-wheat English muffin
- Buckwheat pancakes
- Wild rice pilaf
- Vegetable-stuffed corn tortilla
- Black bean quinoa salad
- Baked corn tortilla chips and salsa
- Whole-grain flours, like whole wheat, as a substitute for a quarter to half of the white flour in recipes
- Whole cornmeal cornbread
- Whole-grain muffins with pumpkin seeds
- Oatmeal cookies

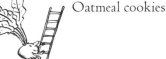

## Get Smart's Nutrition Prescription for Healthy Carbohydrates

| Instead of | Choose |
|---|---|
| White bread | 100% whole-grain bread |
| White rice | Brown or wild rices |
| White pasta | Whole-grain pasta |
| Sugar-coated, refined cereals | Whole-grain cereals (e.g., shredded wheat, oatmeal, Kashi) |
| Chocolate chip cookies | Chocolate chip cookies made with whole-wheat pastry flour, vegan margarine, organic dark chocolate chips |
| Sweetened beverages | Flavored seltzers, tea, water |
| Regular crackers | Whole multigrain crackers |

### Brown Does Not Mean "Whole"

*Pumpernickel, rye, and other darker colored breads are not necessarily made with whole grains. The rye bread I loved as a kid was a blend of white flour and refined rye flour with added caraway seeds. I just spotted a whole-grain rye at Trader Joe's. American-style pumpernickel bread is dark usually because it is colored with molasses, coffee, or chocolate, and it does not contain whole grains.*

*Traditional German pumpernickel is usually made with whole grains.*

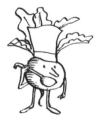

☞ The glycemic index is a measure of the effect of specific foods on blood sugar.

☞ High-glycemic foods means that food—for example, a piece of white bread—causes a fast, big rise in blood sugar levels.

☞ Low-glycemic foods cause a slower, less pronounced rise in blood sugar.

☞ The glycemic load is a cousin of the glycemic index and is too annoying and complicated to explain.

☞ Whole grains are the way to go.

☞ Once in a while eating some white rice or pasta is fine.

I invited my friend Cynthia over for dinner to have farm-fresh zucchini, basil, and tofu on whole-grain pasta. She arrived with a package of her own regular white spaghetti, saying she did not like whole-wheat pasta. Of course I substituted whole-grain pasta for the white stuff, and she couldn't tell the difference. Sometimes the different color bothers people more than the taste. A fun trick with children who are resistant to whole-grain breads is to make a sandwich with half white and half whole-grain breads and cut them into fun shapes.

## Fruit and Vegetable Nirvana

Vegetables and fruits are the beautifying, disease-fighting, antiaging, brain-boosting magical fountain of youth. If you consume them every day, you will be granted eternal life, great prosperity, and full immunity on Project Runway. Perhaps I exaggerate ever so slightly. The Project Runway judges are awfully tough.

### Eat Your Peas and Carrots

I was a guest on the revival of the *Phil Donahue Show* a few years back doing a segment on the dangers of diet pills. On the air Mr. Donahue turned to me and said, "Miss Heller, how can people lose weight? And don't tell us 'eat your peas and carrots.' We already know that." He's right, of course. You know vegetables and fruits are good for you. So why aren't you eating them? The Centers for Disease Control and Prevention report that only 22.1 percent of men and 32.2 percent of women are eating their vegetables. This means that most American brains are not getting the antioxidants they need to slow brain aging and help prevent cognitive decline.

### Live Long and Prosper

*In the European Prospective Investigation of Cancer—Norfolk study, researchers found that the consumption of fruits and vegetables was associated with a substantially decreased risk of diabetes. In another arm of the same study researchers discovered that fruit and vegetable consumption was associated with a lower risk of mortality. So eat fruits and vegetables every day and you'll live a healthier, longer life. It's that simple.*

Donna told me she couldn't stand vegetables.
"How about carrots?" I asked.
"Oh," she replied, "I do like carrots."
"And spinach?"
"Yes I like spinach, too."
"What about broccoli?"
"I'm not sure. I don't remember the last time I ate broccoli. I don't think I liked it."

As time passed and Donna was reintroduced to vegetables, she found many vegetables that she did like, including broccoli. Donna does not like to cook, so we explored easy ways to add vegetables into her diet. One successful idea was to add extra spinach and other vegetables to a no-cheese vegetable frozen pizza she found at the grocery store before she popped it into the oven. She's lost weight and has created a healthy eating lifestyle that includes vegetables daily and fits in with her work and "I don't cook" lifestyle.

## Dealers and Pushers

I am a hard-core vegetable pusher. The reason is that both fruits and vegetables are jam packed with compounds that promote health and healing, fight disease, help manage weight, and support a healthy brain. There is a huge variety from which to choose, and they are very versatile. There are no bad vegetables or fruits, so knock your socks off. The only caveat is that fruit has many more calories than vegetables, so while you can eat lots of vegetables, it is best to stick to two to three servings of fruit a day. One serving of fruit is one apple, one cup of fruit salad or berries, one orange, and so on.

I did not like vegetables as a child. I don't ever remember eating any. One evening when I was about 6 or 7, my mom told me I could not leave the dinner table until I had eaten my peas. I hated peas. In a stroke of what I thought was brilliance, I took the peas and put them in my milk. The white plastic glass filled with milk, I thought, was a perfect hiding place for the peas. "I'm done, Mom," I called, certain that my ruse would work. She came to the table, looked at my plate, then at the glass of milk with the peas in it, and said, "Now, drink your milk, Sam."

---

Eating fruits and vegetables daily will give your body a hefty dose of vitamins, minerals, phytochemicals, and fiber, all of which are essential for a healthy brain and body. Vegetables are low in calories but high in taste and fiber, so you can eat lots of them. In the DASH Diet the U.S. Department of Health and Human Services recommends eating 5–10 servings of fruits and vegetables every day. One serving of vegetables is ½ cup cooked or 1 cup raw. I'd stick with 2–3 fruits a day and fill the rest with vegetables.

## **Your Brain on Fruits and Vegetables**

Fruits and vegetables contain compounds that reduce oxidative stress. Oxidative stress is a normal physiological process that produces free radicals, or oxidants. Oxidative stress becomes harmful when free-radical molecules outnumber the antioxidants and ultimately cause cell damage. Oxidative stress is implicated in the development and progression of brain aging, cognitive decline, and Alzheimer's disease. One of the hallmarks of Alzheimer's disease and other forms of dementia is neurofibrillary tangles and β-amyloid plaques that build up in the brain. Neurofibrillary tangles are abnormal tangles of fibers found inside brain cells. β-amyloid plaques are formed from protein fragments that accumulate between neurons in the brain. In a healthy brain the protein fragments are broken down and eliminated. In a person with Alzheimer's disease they build up and turn into hardened plaques in brain tissue and interfere with the brain's ability to function. Scientists believe that oxidative stress contributes to the formation of neurofibrillary tangles and amyloid plaques. Eating lots of fruits and vegetables helps keep a good supply of antioxidants available to neutralize free radicals, reduce oxidative stress, protect cells, and support a healthy brain and may offer protection against dementia. In the Nurses' Health Study researchers discovered that women who ate the most vegetables, especially green leafy vegetables, had a slower rate of cognitive decline and less decline than women who weren't eating many vegetables. What can I say? Eat your peas and carrots.

 Fruits and vegetables contain antioxidants that help protect the cells and neurons in the brain and the rest of the body.

Vegetables and fruit are also huge contributors of vitamins, minerals, fiber, healthy fats, and phytochemicals, all of which are essential for a well-functioning body. These compounds work synergistically to facilitate and optimize everything from neurons communicating in the brain, muscle function, cardiovascular health, wound healing, skin growth and repair, and disease fighting to regulating mood, appetite, and energy levels. We have the research to show that people who eat a more plant-based diet (meaning lots of fruits and vegetables, whole grains, beans, nuts) have a decreased risk of dementia, cardiovascular disease, and diabetes; they live longer, manage weight better, have lower LDL (bad) cholesterol, and make more money than the people who eat traditional Western diets. The traditional Western diet is generally

## Phamous Phytochemicals from Phruits and Vegetables

| Phytochemical | Food | Potential Benefit |
|---|---|---|
| Beta carotene | carrots, pumpkin, sweet potato, cantaloupe | neutralizes free radicals, which may damage cells; bolsters cellular antioxidant defenses; can be made into vitamin A in the body |
| Lutein, Zeaxanthin | kale, collards, spinach, corn, eggs, citrus | may contribute to maintenance of healthy vision |
| Lycopene | tomatoes and processed tomato products, watermelon, red/pink grapefruit | may contribute to maintenance of prostate health |
| Anthocyanins | berries, cherries, red grapes | bolsters cellular antioxidant defenses; may contribute to maintenance of brain function |
| Flavanols— Catechins, Epicatechins, Epigallocatechin, Procyanidins | tea, cocoa, chocolate, apples, grapes | may contribute to maintenance of heart health |
| Flavonols— Quercetin, Kaempferol, Isorhamnetin, Myricetin | onions, apples, tea, broccoli | neutralize free radicals, which may damage cells; bolster cellular antioxidant defenses |
| Isothiocyanates | cauliflower, broccoli, broccoli sprouts, cabbage, kale, horse-radish | may enhance detoxification of undesirable compounds; bolsters cellular antioxidant defenses |

*Source:* International Food Information Council Foundation, Functional Foods, July 2006, www.ific
.org/nutrition/functional/upload/functionalfoodsbackgrounder.pdf.

considered to consist of red and processed meats, pork, refined carbohydrates, sodas, cheese, fast food, french fries, and desserts.

A more plant-based diet may not increase your earning power. But
there is a good chance it will help you a live a longer, healthier life so
you can enjoy what you do have!

☞   Fruits and vegetables are chock a block full of antioxidants, vitamins, minerals, and phytochemicals that help reduce oxidative stress.

☞   Oxidative stress increases brain aging and cognitive decline.

### Sugar Morph

*Sugar comes in several forms. Glucose and fructose are single players. Other sugars such as sucrose are combinations of sugars. Note how glucose is in all of these combos:*

|  |  |  |
|---|---|---|
| *Maltose* | = | *glucose-glucose* |
| *Sucrose (table sugar)* | = | *fructose-glucose* |
| *Lactose (milk sugar)* | = | *galactose-glucose* |
| *Honey* | = | *glucose-fructose* |

## Carb o' Myths

Let's bust some hardy, long-lasting carbohydrate myths.

### Carbohydrates Make You Fat

No, no, and may I say no. Every food can make you fat if you eat more than your body needs. You can gain or lose weight eating junky food or healthy food. In this instance it is all about calories. Many of us consume a lot of bread, pasta, sweets, sodas, and snack foods. It is easy to gain weight eating refined, processed carbohydrates like these. They taste good and also cause the sugar wave that makes us want to eat more junky food. By lowering your consumption of these foods and switching over to whole grains, dumping the junky snacks and sweets, you will be lowering the amount of carbohydrates you eat daily and you may drop some pounds.

## Carrots Are High in Sugar

I am not sure how this myth got started. Maybe because carrots are sweet. Carrots are not high in sugar and rank low on the glycemic load. Half a cup of raw carrots rates a score of 5 on the glycemic load. Anything less than 10 is considered "low."

Carrots are good for your eyes and other organs because they are high in the antioxidant beta carotene. When I was in college, I took many dance classes and ate a lot of carrots because that is what dancers did. They ate carrots in place of higher-calorie foods to stay thin. I ate so many carrots that eventually the palms of my hands turned an orangey yellow color from all the beta carotene in the carrots—a clear sign I needed some variety in my vegetable intake.

## Satan's Temptation

Sugar is not the Antichrist. It feeds your brain and your cells. Sugar is thought of as sinful because it is usually tied up with junky foods like cookies, cakes, ice cream, deep-fried Twinkies (what diabolical mind came up with that idea?), sweetened beverages, candy, and other non-nutritive, high-calorie foods. It makes sense to limit foods high in sugar because they are also high in calories, usually contain bad fat, have virtually no health benefits, and wreak havoc with blood sugar levels. That said, adding some sugar to your coffee or indulging in a small fat-free frozen yogurt will not land you in purgatory.

## Sugar Causes Diabetes

It seems logical to think that eating sugary foods causes diabetes, since diabetes is a blood sugar problem. In fact, obesity is one of the strongest predictors of type 2 diabetes. Abdominal obesity, fat around your middle, increases the risk even more. People whose diets are high in refined carbohydrates, bad saturated fat, and animal foods and who do not exercise are at an increased risk of developing type 2 diabetes.

## Honey Is Better for You Than Sugar

**Honeybee Fact:**
Let's save our
honeybees by using
fewer pesticides
and reducing global
warming, two
possible reasons for
the decline in the
honeybee population.

If you think honey is better for you than sugar because it is not white table sugar, think again. "I don't eat sugar," Keri said smugly. "I just use honey." How, I wondered, can I break the news to her that honey is pretty much metabolized the same way regular sugar is?

Generally speaking, all carbohydrates lead to glucose. Honey is made up of glucose and fructose and an enzyme called glucose oxidase. Fructose is metabolized a bit differently, but most of our dietary carbohydrates like pasta and honey become glucose in the body. Molasses, rice syrup, honey, "raw" sugar, brown sugar, and agave nectar are all forms of sugar and are metabolized pretty much the same way in the body.

Honey is cool because it has been used for centuries as a healing tonic and balm in folk medicine. It contains antioxidants that help protect cells. Used topically, honey is effective in wound dressings that are used to treat burns, wounds, and infections. In July 2007 the Food and Drug Administration gave honey the nod and approved the use of honey-based wound dressings in the United States. The sugar content of honey keeps microorganisms from growing, and glucose oxidase produces hydrogen peroxide that provides direct antibacterial protection. Amazing what bees can do.

## High-Fructose Corn Syrup Makes You Fat

There are two questions everyone asks about high-fructose corn syrup. Is high-fructose corn syrup (HFCS) really all natural? And does it make you fat? The easy answer to the first question is "no." HFCS is not found in nature as HFCS. Originally HFCS comes from corn starch. The chemical structure is altered by changing the original glucose that comes from the starch over to fructose. Fructose is a naturally occurring sugar found in fruits and vegetables. The newly created fructose is then added to corn syrup to create the now ubiquitous HFCS. HFCS is a cheaper alternative to cane or beet sugar. HFCS is found in everything including soda, bread, frozen desserts, salad dressing, jam, cereal, and ketchup. A study in the *American Journal of Clinical Nutrition* reported an increase in the consumption of HFCS of more than 1,000 percent between 1970 and 2000 in the United States. Another survey of more than

21,000 children and adults found that 74 percent of the fructose in their diet came from sugar-sweetened beverages and other processed foods (unfortunately, it did not come from fruits and vegetables).

But does HFCS make you fat? Technically no, since HFCS is pretty similar on the molecular level to regular sugar and it does not magically pack on the pounds. There is controversy surrounding the effects of HFCS on weight gain. One reason is that HFCS is in foods that are associated with weight gain, such as sugar-sweetened beverages (SSBs) like soda and fruit drinks. An analysis examining children's consumption of sugar-sweetened beverages found a significant relationship between kids who drink a lot of SSBs and their body mass index—meaning they are getting fat. The same goes for women who drink sugar-sweetened beverages. The Nurses' Health Study found that frequent consumption of SSBs is associated with greater weight gain and an increased risk for type 2 diabetes and coronary heart disease in women. Other studies have shown a parallel rise in the consumption of HFCS and the staggering increase in obesity and type 2 diabetes in the United States. Of concern also is that the body processes fructose differently than glucose and because of this may bypass the body's ability to regulate feelings of hunger and fullness, so we eat more. Finally some research is showing that fructose increases inflammatory markers, triglycerides, and abdominal fat. The bottom line is that because HFCS is found in so many processed foods and beverages and we are eating far too many of these foods, we, as a nation, are gaining weight and getting sick. Naturally occurring fructose, which is found in fruits and vegetables, comes in small quantities and can be consumed without concern. But foods we eat that have added fructose and HFCS, like SSBs, fast food, and junk food, should be limited.

P.S. Do not be fooled by the food industry replacing HFCS with sucrose (sugar) in processed foods and beverages. If you eat a lot of these, you will still gain weight.

**Lactose Fact:** People who are lactose intolerant do not have the enzyme in their gut that helps digest lactose, called lactase. Lactase helps break apart the galactose-glucose molecule so it can be absorbed. If you do not have the enzyme lactase in your gut, eating dairy products may cause cramping or bloating.

## Sweet Memories

Glucose appears to play a significant role in memory and cognition. No one knows exactly why yet, but researchers speculate that it is partly because glucose is a fuel source and partly because glucose is a precursor to acetylcholine, a neurotransmitter that plays roles in learning and memory. Studies of the effects of glucose, from either food like a potato or a glucose (sugary) drink, have been done with young, elderly, and military folk. Overall the results indicate that consuming glucose improves vigilance, memory, mood, and learning. If you have not eaten in a while and need a brain boost, chow down on a carbohydrate combined with some protein. The carbohydrate will give your brain a boost, and the protein will help regulate energy levels.

## Muffins and Matchmakers

Studies show that eating carbohydrates helps boost brain function. A study in the *American Journal of Clinical Nutrition* found that feeding carbohydrates (in this case in the form of potatoes and barley) to subjects with poor memories enhanced their cognition. I have noticed with my mother that often, though not always, after she eats she becomes more focused and has less trouble finding words. A case in point: It was a lovely summer's day, so I took my mother to the courtyard of her nursing home, where we could sit under a tree and she could eat her corn muffin. Some of the staff was setting up in the courtyard for a small outdoor barbeque. We were sitting a few feet away from the grill. The chef came out and started grilling hot dogs and hamburgers. As Mom and I got up to leave, the chef and I starting chatting. I told him I was a dietitian, and he was telling me about the company he works for.

"Mom," I said, "he is a chef here. He makes the recipes and prepares the food in the café."

"Oh," she replied, interested.

"Yes," the chef said. "My family and friends are always happy when there is party so I can do the cooking!"

"Well," replied Mom, "we will just have to be at the next one."

The chef looked at me, perplexed.

"She just invited us to your next party," I told him.

Mom stood for a bit and tried to continue the conversation with the chef as best she could. After a bit of prodding I finally got her to come inside.

"He was cute," she pointed out.

"Yes, Mom . . ." I stopped and looked at her. "Oh my God, you were trying to get him to ask me out, weren't you?"

"Well," she replied slyly, "it couldn't hurt."

Amazing what a corn muffin can do.

## Brain-Boosting Snacks

- Apple and low-fat cheese
- Whole-grain cracker (like Rvita or Wasa) with a schmeer of cashew butter (about 2 teaspoons) and topped with sliced strawberries
- ½ sliced banana in 1 cup fat-free plain yogurt, with a dash of cinnamon
- the classic: ½ cup low-fat cottage cheese and ¼ sliced cantaloupe or honeydew melon
- 2 figs (fresh or dried) sliced and topped with a few walnuts halves (I like figs dipped in tahini, a sesame paste that makes great dips and salad dressings, with a few drops of honey)

## The Sugar Whos?

As early as 1922, scientists noticed that people with type 1 and type 2 diabetes suffered from impaired memory and attention. We now know that diabetes is a risk factor for dementia and cognitive decline. The reasons are varied and not completely understood, but scientists think that cardiovascular disease associated with diabetes, chronic high blood sugar, and oxidative stress plays a part in the relationship between diabetes and cognitive function. It is worth mentioning because in 2008 the Centers for Disease Control and Prevention estimated that 24 million people in the United States had diabetes and that another 57 million people were prediabetic, and according to the National Institutes of Health, approximately 6 million people have diabetes but don't know it. It is a safe bet that someone reading this book is in one of those categories.

## What to Do

See your physician and find out if you are prediabetic or have metabolic syndrome or diabetes. If you have any of these conditions, it is critical that you take action immediately. Consult a registered dietitian or certified diabetes educator to help teach you what you need to know about healthy eating and lifestyle changes. Healthy eating plans like *Get Smart*'s Nutrition Prescription will help you reduce the risk of developing diabetes if you are prediabetic, manage the disease if you are a diagnosed diabetic, and lower the risk of developing cardiovascular disease, stroke, hypertension, dementia, and other complications associated with diabetes.

Diabetes is a very serious disease and has reached epic proportions in the United States and around the world. Diabetes significantly increases the risk of cognitive decline and dementia. Even prediabetes or metabolic syndrome are risk factors for brain dysfunction. It is never too late to adopt a healthy lifestyle to help manage diabetes and help regain your brain and physical health.

## The Sugar Blues: Diabetes

The American Diabetes Association defines diabetes mellitus as a group of metabolic diseases characterized by hyperglycemia (high levels of blood glucose) resulting from defects in insulin secretion, insulin action, or both. The chronic hyperglycemia of diabetes is associated with long-term damage, dysfunction, and failure of various organs, especially the eyes, kidneys, nerves, heart, and blood vessels.

If you have type 2 diabetes, it means your body is having a tough time getting the glucose or blood sugar out of the arteries and into the cells. You might be resistant to the effects of insulin or not be producing enough insulin to handle a glucose load after a meal. Type 1 diabetes means that your pancreas is not producing any insulin due to a variety of possible reasons, including viral or genetic influences.

## Metabolic Syndrome

Metabolic syndrome puts you at serious risk of developing type 2 diabetes and cardiovascular disease. Metabolic syndrome is defined by the National Cholesterol Education Program as the presence of any three of the following conditions:

- Excess weight around the waist (waist measurement of more than 40 inches for men and more than 35 inches for women)
- High levels of triglycerides (150 mg/dL or higher)
- Low levels of HDL, or "good," cholesterol (below 40 mg/dL for men and below 50 mg/dL for women)
- High blood pressure (130/85 mm Hg or higher)
- High fasting blood glucose levels (110 mg/dL or higher)

## Prediabetes

The Centers for Disease Control and Prevention identify prediabetes as blood sugars that are higher than normal but not yet in the diabetic range. If you have prediabetes, you are in luck because with healthy lifestyle changes including diet and exercise you can dodge the path to developing full-blown type 2 diabetes.

☞  Glucose boosts memory and learning.

☞  Diabetes is a disorder that affects how well your body handles glucose and insulin.

☞  Diabetes is a risk factor for dementia and cognitive decline as well as cardiovascular disease.

☞  See your physician to find out if you are at risk of developing diabetes.

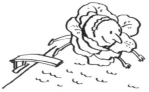

- Carbohydrates get broken down into glucose in the body.
- Glucose is the primary and preferred source of fuel for your brain and working muscles.
- Insulin is necessary to get glucose out of the arteries and into the cells, where it is used for energy and fuel.
- Refined carbohydrates, aka junky carbohydrates, such as pretzels, muffins, Italian bread, candy, and sweetened beverages like sodas and fruit drinks, play havoc with the body's ability to manage blood sugar levels.
- Regular consumption of junky carbohydrates increases the risk of developing type 2 diabetes, cardiovascular disease, cognitive decline, metabolic syndrome, and obesity.
- Whole grains are really good for you and taste good, too.
- Vegetables, fruits, beans, and nuts contain carbohydrates.
- Vegetables and fruits help protect the brain from oxidative damage.
- Most people are not eating enough vegetables and fruits.
- Carbohydrates improve memory, learning, and mood, so be sure to include them with breakfast.

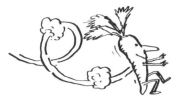

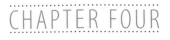
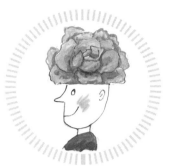

## CHAPTER FOUR

# Your ABCs: Vitamins and Minerals

--- KEY POINTS ---

⇨ Vitamin and mineral supplements should be used sparingly.

⇨ Some supplements are a good idea for brain health.

⇨ B vitamins are big players in the brain.

⇨ Experts warn of widespread vitamin D deficiency.

⇨ Minerals like iron and zinc are necessary for brain development and function.

⇨ Excess sodium can lead to high blood pressure and a decline in cognitive function.

## ────── NUTRITION PRESCRIPTION ──────
### *for* VITAMINS *and* MINERALS

⇨ **Take a multivitamin and vitamin D supplement daily (women should also take calcium supplements).**

⇨ **Eat foods high in B vitamins.**

⇨ **Eat foods high in vitamins C and E.**

### Rhythm 'n' Blues

Every essential vitamin and mineral has indispensable roles in brain function. Like a hot jazz band, vitamins and minerals need each other, everyone on different instruments, some taking solos, some playing more supportive parts, some having an attitude, yet they all work together as an ensemble. Making sure your brain has a balanced band of vitamins and minerals is key for hitting all the right notes.

### Multitasking

Getting the nutrients your brain needs from food is always the first choice, since foods contain an array of healthy compounds that work together. It is well known that children and adults who are well nourished have better cognitive function than those who are not. Vitamin and mineral status is affected by many things, such as illness, lifestyle, age, stress, food availability, and even latitude. Even a slight vitamin deficiency can cause problems. For example:

| Deficiency | *Disease* |
|---|---|
| Vitamin C | *Scurvy* |
| Vitamin D | *Rickets* |
| Thiamin | *Beriberi* |
| Niacin | *Pellagra* |

Most of us are not perfect in our daily dietary choices; our diets often fall short of certain essential vitamins and minerals. For example, the National Institutes of Health warn that most Americans are short on magnesium, and experts suggest that there is a worldwide insufficiency of vitamin D. Taking a multivitamin daily will help fill the gaps in your overall vitamin and mineral levels.

Remember that "supplements" are just what they sound like: supplements to a healthy diet. Washing down a vitamin pill with a soda and an order of fries is counterproductive, to say the least. Megadosing is another no-no. No point in taking tons of a substance when your body can use only a smidgen of it at a time. Overdosing on any single vitamin, mineral, or herb can lead to metabolic imbalances and toxic side effects.

Avoid megadosing with supersupplements or megafortified foods. Some cereals, energy or nutrition bars, and other fortified foods deliver high amounts of vitamins like folate. For example, many fortified cereals have the full recommended 400 micrograms (mcg) of folate. Combine that with a folic-acid-fortified energy bar that has up to 800 mcg of folic acid, and you would be over the limit for the Institute of Medicine's upper limit of 1,000 mcg of folic acid daily from fortified foods. FYI, you won't OD on vitamins and minerals eating whole, healthy foods.

My friend Sarah is a breast cancer survivor. She does not exercise. When we go out to eat, she always has wine and then orders at least two desserts. She slathers white bread with butter. On her summer vacation she was eating pastrami sandwiches, fried clams, and cheese fondue. Sarah carries a bag of supplements, herbs, and green tea bags around with her. She carefully lays out her daily supplement doses and washes them down with green tea. She has heard that green tea is protective against breast cancer. I don't say much to her, since she hasn't asked and is not my patient. It is difficult watching her eat foods—like butter, red meat, and alcohol—that significantly increase her risk of a breast cancer recurrence. I think she feels the pills, herbs, and teas will protect her. But the reality is that the saturated fat, refined foods, lack of exercise, and alcohol intake will do her far more harm than any supplement can help.

Your *Get Smart* Nutrition Prescription is to take a daily multivitamin and a vitamin D supplement.

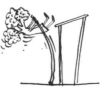

**Multis and You**

- Multivitamin supplement use might reduce the risk of breast cancer among women consuming alcohol or decrease the risk of developing estrogen receptor-progesterone receptor (ER-PR) breast cancer.
- B6, folate, and riboflavin may be protective against colorectal cancer.
- Dietary intake (what you get from food) of folate, B6, and B12 is associated with a reduced risk of heart disease.
- Regular use of multivitamin supplements may decrease the risk of ovulatory infertility.
- Regular vitamin and mineral supplement takers were found to have healthier profiles (e.g., lower homocysteine, lower risk of high blood pressure and diabetes) than non–supplement takers.
- One study found that "excessive use" of multivitamins (more than seven times a week) increased the risk of prostate cancer, especially for those men with a family history of prostate cancer. Regular multivitamin users were not at increased risk. This study generated a lot of press and confusion. The link is not clear or definitive at this point.

## Brainy B Good

We all hope our kids get As in school, but it is the Bs in the brain that help make As on the page possible. There are several B vitamins, and they all work together as a team. They work with many other vitamins, minerals, and compounds in the brain, too. The Bs include niacin, thiamin, B6, B12, folate, riboflavin, pantothenic acid, and biotin. The Bs are water soluble, meaning that if there are Bs in excess of your body's needs, they will be excreted in your urine.

While all the Bs are important in brain function, research has been particularly focused on folate and B12 and their relationship to cognitive function and cardiovascular disease. It is difficult to determine which vitamin does what, when, and in what amounts when it comes to examining their effects on chronic diseases. Even though medical experts do not yet know if taking B supplements makes a difference in dementia or cardiovascular disease risk, the nutrition prescription here is to eat a diet with loads of B foods. You will also get Bs in your multi.

Without a good balance of Bs, the brain band will be hitting sour notes and mangled chords. Get your Bs from food and a multivitamin.

## Homocysteine

Bee-fore we get to the Bs, we need to talk about homocysteine. Homocysteine is an amino acid that is a by-product of normal protein metabolism (metabolism is a series of chemical and physical processes that involves the conversion of food to energy and the use of energy in the body). When the body breaks down certain proteins, it makes homocysteine. High levels of homocysteine in the blood have been linked to cardiovascular disease, stroke, mortality, cognitive decline, and Alzheimer's disease and other forms of dementia. Homocysteine is mentioned here because its metabolism is intimately involved with the Bs. Scientists are looking at the Bs, their relationship with homocysteine,

### Don't Worry, Be Happy

*Is your neighbor's leaf blower annoying you? Are you fantasizing about plowing into the car of the stupid driver who just cut you off? Do you feel like that guy in the 1981 David Cronenberg movie* Scanners? *Where his head blows up? (I saw only the trailer. I can't watch violent movies.) All that hostility could be setting you up for some serious problems. One small study found that hostility was associated with elevated homocysteine levels, which are associated with heart disease and dementia. So head for the sunny side of the street and plaster a big smile on your face.*

and how varying levels of each individually and together affect the risk of Alzheimer's disease and other dementias. They have not figured it all out yet, but there is no doubt that having a good balance of Bs in the body is necessary for a bee-autiful brain.

Homocysteine is a by-product of normal protein metabolism. Too much homocysteine increases the risk of a brain implosion. The Bee-onators keep homocysteine in check.

## The Bee Band Players

In the food recommendations below, I did not include ready-to-eat cereals and many breads, pastas, and flours, since they are fortified with essential vitamins and minerals. Also, many foods have lots of different vitamins; I listed different foods for each vitamin for variety's sake. I included only foods that fit in with *Get Smart*'s Nutrition Prescription recommendations.

Folate

Folate is also known as folic acid. Folic acid is the synthetic form of folate that is used in vitamins and to fortify foods. Low folate levels in the blood have been linked to cognitive decline and Alzheimer's disease and other forms of dementia. Higher levels of folate are associated with better cognitive performance and a lower risk of developing Alzheimer's disease.

The National Academy of Science's 2002 Dietary Reference Intakes (DRI) recommends 400 mcg of folate a day.

**Folate Functions**
- Works with B12 to metabolize homocysteine
- Assists in DNA synthesis
- Is required by rapidly dividing cells such as gastrointestinal tract cells
- Prevents neural tube defects, such as spina bifida, in developing fetuses

| Folate Foods | Amount | Mcg |
|---|---|---|
| Lentils, cooked | 1 cup | 358 |
| Black-eyed peas, cooked | 1 cup | 358 |
| Okra, frozen-cooked | 1 cup | 269 |
| Spinach, cooked | 1 cup | 263 |
| Asparagus, cooked | 4 spears | 89 |
| Collards, cooked | 1 cup | 177 |
| Broccoli, cooked | 1 cup | 168 |
| Papaya, raw | 1 fruit | 116 |
| Romaine lettuce | 1 cup | 76 |
| Orange | 1 fruit | 39 |
| Strawberries | 1 cup | 40 |

**Folate Study Fact:** Epidemiological studies (studies that look at large groups of people) suggest a relationship between folate, homocysteine, and hearing loss. One study done in the Netherlands before folic acid supplementation was common in foods found that folic acid supplementation seemed to slow the decline of low-frequency hearing loss in folate-deficient, older adults.

## Heavy Metal Meets the B12 Blues: B12

Vitamin B12 is primarily found in animal foods and is also in fortified foods like fortified cereals. B12 contains the metal cobalt, so it is also known as cobalamine. Low vitamin B12 levels are associated with cognitive decline, impairment, depression, and dementia. There is a chemical in the stomach called intrinsic factor that binds to B12 and helps absorption. As we get older, we tend to have less of this chemical, so we absorb less vitamin B12. People over 65 are at risk of low vitamin B12 levels and should consider taking a vitamin B12 supplement.

I was at an antique store in the Pocono Mountains eyeing some cobalt blue milk bottles and was asking the dealer about them. I have always loved cobalt blue glassware. "Yep," he said. "The ladies always go for the cobalt glassware. Not the men though." He had no idea why. You can buy cobalt blue glassware for fun, but it does not supply any B12! You have to get that from food.

The 2002 DRI recommends 2.4 mcg of vitamin B12 a day.

### B12 Functions
- Helps maintain healthy nerve cells
- Is necessary for folate absorption
- Assists in DNA synthesis
- Is required by rapidly dividing cells, such as those in the intestinal tract, respiratory tract, and bone marrow

- Works with folate to reduce levels of homocysteine

| Vitamin B12 Foods | Amount | Mcg |
|---|---|---|
| Chicken, cooked | 1 cup | 13.69 |
| Sardines, canned in oil | 3 oz | 7.6 |
| Trout, rainbow, cooked | 3 oz | 4.22 |
| Fat-free milk | 1 cup | 1.3 |
| Low-fat yogurt | 8 oz | 1.27 |
| Fried egg | 1 | 0.64 |
| Low-fat cottage cheese | 1 cup | 1.42 |
| Low-fat Swiss cheese | 1 slice | 2.0 |

*I was doing a TV show and a guest host asked me whether she should continue getting B12 shots. I asked her why she was getting them. She thought they gave her energy. Contrary to popular belief, vitamin B12 does not give you energy. A deficiency of B12 can lead to anemia and fatigue. However, if you do not have a deficiency of vitamin B12, shots of it won't pump up your perk. If you are suffering from a vitamin B12 deficiency, supplementation is a reasonable option. But you also need to find out why there is a deficiency.*

*Since vegetarians and especially vegans (vegans are vegetarians who go one step further and do not eat dairy) do not eat much, if any, animal foods, they need to be sure they are getting B12 from either supplements, low-fat or nonfat dairy foods, or fortified foods.*

## Sittin' in with Niacin: B3

Few studies have looked at whether dietary niacin (how much niacin you get in food each day) affects the risk of cognitive decline. In one study researchers found that people who had diets high in niacin had a decreased risk of Alzheimer's disease and cognitive decline. Even though this is only one study looking specifically at niacin and Alzheimer's disease, there have been many others examining dietary Bs that show that the Bs have a significant effect on brain function. In fact, symptoms of pellagra, the disease caused by niacin deficiency, include dementia, confusion, and disorientation. Common sense tells us that keeping adequate amounts of niacin in our brain is a darn good idea.

The 2002 DRI recommends 14 mg of niacin a day for women, 16 mg a day for men.

### Niacin Functions

- Assists in the metabolism of fat, carbohydrate, and protein
- Is unique because it is the only B vitamin that can be made from the amino acid tryptophan
- Raises HDL cholesterol (good) levels
- Is important for healthy skin, hair, eyes, and digestive system

| Niacin Foods | Amount | Mg |
| --- | --- | --- |
| Tuna, light, canned | 3 oz | 11.28 |
| Chicken breast, roasted | ½ breast | 14.73 |
| Mushrooms, cooked | 1 cup | 7.0 |
| Peanuts, dry roasted (no salt) | 1 oz (28 peanuts) | 3.8 |
| Pearled barley, cooked | 1 cup | 3.2 |
| Brown rice, cooked | 1 cup | 3.0 |
| Peas, green, frozen, boiled | 1 cup | 2.36 |
| Parsnips, cooked, boiled | 1 cup | 1.13 |

## Roll over Bee-thoven: Thiamin (B1)

When I was little, my older sister told me if I wasn't careful I would get beriberi and die. I thought she meant Chuck Berry. You have to cut me some slack here. I was very young, and my siblings are older than I, and I believed everything they told me. Beriberi was first written about in the early sixteenth century in the Far East. Initially beriberi was thought to be caused by a bacterium or virus. It took centuries for scientists to figure out that beriberi was caused by a deficiency that was related to the consumption of white rice, a staple in the Asian diet. When white rice is polished, the bran and the embryo of the grain are removed, taking virtually all the vitamins, minerals, fats, and protein with them, including thiamin. Researchers eventually made the connection between polished white rice and the onset of beriberi but still did not know the exact cause. It took many more years before thiamin was discovered and used to cure beriberi. Ultimately, this discovery led to the act of enriching white rice and white flour with B vitamins, iron, and other compounds to avoid deficiencies.

Clinical signs of thiamin deficiency include apathy, decreased memory, confusion, and irritability. In today's world, in Western societies, the main group at risk of thiamin deficiency is people who regularly consume excessive alcohol. This may be due to poor diet or the effect alcohol has on thiamin absorption and utilization. As we age, thiamin levels tend to decrease, also.

The 2002 DRI recommends 1.1 mg of thiamin a day for women, 1.2 mg a day for men.

### Thiamin Functions
- Contributes to nerve and muscle health
- Assists in the metabolism of energy

| Thiamin Foods | Amount | Mg |
|---|---|---|
| Pinto beans, cooked | 1 cup | 0.33 |
| Pistachios, dry roasted | 1 oz (47 nuts) | 0.24 |
| Orange juice | 1 cup | 0.22 |
| Tahini | 1 tbs | 0.18 |
| Oat bran muffin | 1 | 0.15 |
| Mango | 1 | 0.12 |

## Bee Sharp with B6: Pyridoxine

Vitamin B6, also known as pyridoxine, facilitates more than 100 chemical reactions. Deficiencies are rarely seen in the United States, but many older folks have low blood levels of B6, which may contribute to depression and confusion.

The 2002 DRI recommends 1.3 mg of vitamin B6 a day; for those over 50: 1.5 mg a day for women, 1.7 mg a day for men.

**Vitamin B6 Functions**
- Assists in the metabolism of amino acid, glucose, fat, and homocysteine
- Contributes to neurotransmitter production
- Assists in DNA and RNA synthesis

| Vitamin B6 Foods | Amount | Mg |
|---|---|---|
| Chickpeas (garbanzo beans), cooked | 1 cup | 1.13 |
| Roasted chestnuts | 1 cup | 0.7 |
| Prune juice, canned | 1 cup | 0.56 |
| Banana | 1 | 0.43 |
| Sweet potato, canned | 1 cup | 0.48 |
| Brussels sprouts, frozen, cooked | 1 cup | 0.45 |
| Potato, boiled, with skin | 1 potato | 0.42 |
| Plantains, cooked | 1 cup | 0.37 |
| Refried beans, canned | 1 cup | 0.36 |
| Halibut, broiled | 3 oz | 0.34 |
| Turnip greens, boiled | 1 cup | 0.26 |

Patty's dad had Alzheimer's. She was visiting him one day. He was trying to communicate something to her, but she was having trouble figuring it out. "Piggys," he said. "Piggies." Then, "Cu . . . cu . . . cucumbers."

Patty repeated what he had said: "OK, Dad, piggies and cucumbers. What about them?"

"*Piggies,*" he insisted. Patty thought about this for a minute. "If I didn't know him so well, I would not have figured it out," she told me. "His feet were cold. Piggies as in 'This little Piggy went to market,' a child's game played with toes. And cucumbers, as in the saying 'cold as a cucumber.'"

Makes perfect sense to me.

## D-ivas, C-oluraturas, and E-flats: The Other Vitamin Players

### Dee-Light-Ful: Vitamin D

Vitamin D is called the sunshine vitamin because the sun's rays stimulate vitamin D production in the skin. Vitamin D is critical for healthy bones, muscles, immune system, and the metabolism of calcium and phosphorous. Low levels of vitamin D are associated with depression and cognitive impairment.

Most of us are not getting enough vitamin D. In fact, scientists warn of a vitamin D deficiency in the general public. It has been estimated that 1 billion people worldwide have vitamin D deficiency or insufficiency. Those at particular risk are people who live in northern latitudes, elderly people, pregnant women, vegans, and the obese. If you live north of the latitude of Atlanta, Georgia, the sun is not strong enough to stimulate vitamin D production in skin from October to March. When spring comes and the sun's strength increases or if you live south of latitude 33.78, you should be wearing sunscreen to prevent skin cancer. Sunscreen blocks harmful ultraviolet rays but also diminishes the skin's ability to produce vitamin D.

Vitamin D is found in oily fish such as mackerel, sardines, and salmon; fortified ready-to-eat cereals; and milk. It is difficult to get all the D we need from food, so vitamin D supplements are recommended. Most vitamin pills contain about 400 IU (international units) of vitamin D. Experts suggest doubling that to at least 800–1,000 IU of vitamin D daily. Too much of a good thing is too much of a good thing, so don't go overboard with D supplementation. Vitamin D is fat soluble, meaning if you take too much it can become toxic. Get your Ds with supplements, fortified foods, low-fat dairy, and sunshine.

The 2002 DRI recommends 400 IU of vitamin D a day (but that recommendation will change soon).

### Vitamin D Functions
- Contributes to healthy bones, muscles
- Strengthens immune system
- Assists in the metabolism of calcium and phosphorous

---

### Energizer D-ee

*The research on vitamin D just keeps going and going. Vitamin D may be protective against cancers including colon and breast, may decrease the risk of fractures, metabolic syndrome, and type 2 diabetes, and has been linked with a reduced incidence of multiple sclerosis. Low vitamin D levels have been associated with an increased risk of cardiovascular disease, all-cause mortality, glucose intolerance, high blood pressure, and some infectious diseases.*

---

## The Rarest Animal of All

"PUSHMI-PULLYUS are now extinct. That means, there aren't any more. But long ago, when Doctor Dolittle was alive, there were some of them still left in the deepest jungles of Africa; and even then they were very, very scarce. They had no tail, but a head at each end, and sharp horns on each head."

With a head on each end, there was always a game of pushme–pullyou going on. Hugh Lofting wrote about the elusive Pushmi-Pullyus in his books chronicling Dr. Doolittle's world adventures in *The Story of Dr. Doolittle* series.

There is not such creative whimsy in the world of scientific research, but there is certainly a lot of pushme-pullyou going on. In this case, since we are in the vitamin chapter, I refer to the studies being done on the vitamins C and E. Vitamins C and E are powerful antioxidants and work well in tandem to quench free radicals and protect cells from oxidative damage. Since oxidative stress is such a concern for cognitive decline, it is not surprising that scientists are doing studies to see how these vitamins affect the brain. Dietary vitamin C or E means how much of these vitamins people are getting in their diet. Supplemental means taking C and E as vitamin pills. Studies looking at the dietary or supplemental intakes of vitamins C and E have conflicting results. Some studies found that eating or taking vitamins C and E reduced the risk of development of Alzheimer's and other dementias, and others found no relationship. This is a perfect example of the push me–pull you syndrome. Have no fear—your nutrition prescription will set you in the right direction: eat foods high in vitamins C and E for brain health and because these foods also have a lot of other vitamins, minerals, and phytochemicals that your brain and body need.

## Hitting High C: Ascorbic Acid

**Vitamin C Fact:**
Eating fruits and vegetables high in vitamin C helps reduce the risk of developing type 2 diabetes. Eat oranges, broccoli, papaya, and cauliflower. Delish!

Nobel Prize–winning scientist Linus Pauling helped make vitamin C a star. Vitamin C is famous for its powerful antioxidant and immune-boosting skills. In 1970 Pauling's book *Vitamin C and the Common Cold* suggested that high doses of vitamin C could help cure the common cold. Since then people have been megadosing with vitamin C as a cure-all for just about everything from cancer to the flu. To date there is no scientific evidence that megadosing with vitamin C prevents colds, cancer, or the flu. Certainly vitamin C is critical for total body health as well as brain health, but you have to be careful not to oversaturate yourself with C.

The 2002 DRI recommends 75 mg of vitamin C a day for women, 90 mg a day for men.

### Vitamin C Functions
- Assists in collagen synthesis and formation
- Is a powerful antioxidant
- Helps wound healing
- Is a structural component of blood vessels, tendons, ligaments, and bone
- Takes part in the synthesis of the neurotransmitter, norepinephrine

| Vitamin C Foods | Amount | Mg |
|---|---|---|
| Peaches, frozen, sliced | 1 cup | 235.5 |
| Red peppers, sweet, raw | 1 cup | 190.3 |
| Cranberry juice | 8 oz | 107 |
| Pink grapefruit juice | 1 cup | 94 |
| Pineapple, raw | 1 cup | 74 |
| Kiwi | 1 | 70.5 |

| | | |
|---|---|---|
| Cauliflower, frozen, cooked | 1 cup | 56.3 |
| Kale, cooked, boiled | 1 cup | 53.3 |
| Cabbage, Chinese, cooked, boiled | 1 cup | 44.2 |
| Beet greens, cooked, boiled | 1 cup | 36 |
| Melon, honeydew | 1 cup | 30.6 |

## You Scurvy Dog!

*Long ago men sailed the sea for mystery and adventure. They followed their dreams into the navy, to ferry cargo, and for exploration. As far back as 1496, when Vasco da Gama's ships sailed to India, sailors reported coming down with a dreaded disease while at sea. It was described by a Portuguese poet as an affliction of swollen gums and putrid smells. History claims that almost all of Magellan's crew suffered from this horrible disease, but no one knew what it was. In 1753 a British physician named James Lind wrote a treatise describing the causes and cure of what he called scurvy. With no refrigeration, fruits and vegetables would go bad quickly at sea. For months on end sailors had no source of vitamin C, which, Lind figured out, was the cause of scurvy. Red tape being the same then as now, it took many years before the British Admiralty officially approved the use of lemons on ships. At one point sailors tried using limes, which were less expensive, as their source of vitamin C and were called Limeys. The limes did not pack the vitamin C punch they needed, so lemons were reinstated, but the name Limey, referring to British sailors, stuck.*

## The Key of E: Vitamin E (alpha-tocopherol)

Vitamin E is well known too. E works in concert with C to create a potent defense against free radicals and oxidative damage. Vitamin E is fat-soluble, which means that you should eat your vitamin E food with some healthy fats (like olive oil) for optimal absorption.

The 2002 DRI recommends 15 mg of vitamin E a day (= 22.5 IU).

### Vitamin E Functions
- Is a strong antioxidant
- Assists in DNA repair
- Aids in immune system function

| Vitamin E Foods | Amount | Mg |
|---|---|---|
| Sunflower seeds, dry roasted | ¼ cup | 8.35 |
| Spinach, cooked | 1 cup | 3.74 |
| Peanut oil | 1 tbs | 2.12 |
| Beans, white, boiled | 1 cup | 2.1 |
| Chocolate éclair | 1 | 2.01 |
| (Just wanted to see if you were paying attention) | | |
| Raspberries, frozen, red | 1 cup | 1.8 |
| Tortilla chips, corn, white | 1 oz | 1.22 |
| Wheat germ, toasted | 1 tbs | 1.14 |
| Carrots, raw | 1 cup | 0.73 |
| Avocado | 1 oz | 0.75 |

## Scam-a-Rama

There are thousands of supplements on the market today and new ones popping up all the time. It is virtually impossible for the Federal Trade Commission to investigate every one of them. It is up to you to be an informed and educated consumer. Be wary of sensationalized claims for pills, powders, and potions. Get your health information from health professionals such as registered dietitians, physicians, and nurse practitioners. Unfortunately, some "professionals"—Doctors So-and-So—are selling supplements with crazy claims. Before you spend your hard-earned cash, sit down with your physician or a registered dietitian and find what you really need.

Barbara, a retired woman in her sixties, came to see me with a bag of no fewer than 25 bottles of over-the-counter pills, supplements, and herbs. She was told by a "holistic health physician" that she needed all

## Forget about Magic Memory-, Brain-, and IQ-Boosting Supplements

*There are many supplements on the market today promising improved memory and mental focus. Their ads are seductive and couched in pseudoscientific terms that make them seem believable. The truth is that the claims are not backed up by current science. So fuggedaboudit. Save your money and brain power and buy some broccoli instead.*

*One company selling a memory-boosting supplement asked me to do some consulting work for it. We'll call it Company X. Initially I was asked to compile research on omega-3 fatty acids. Two weeks after I started, the president of Company X asked me to appear in an infomercial selling its brain-boosting supplement. In addition to my concern about the claims the company was making in TV commercials about its supplements, I found that the company had numerous complaints about its business practices. (I Googled the Better Business Bureau along with the company name.) The Company X president asked to meet with me to discuss the infomercial. When I met him and asked about the veracity of the supplement claims and the questionable business practices, he fired me on the spot. Not long after I was canned, Company X was fined $1 million by the Federal Trade Commission for making unsubstantiated advertising claims for its memory-boosting products. May I say "Ha, ha!"*

these pills to prevent a heart attack. He told her she had to buy them from him, and she ended up spending more than $300. I reviewed every bottle, and there were only two that I thought she should keep—a calcium supplement and a multivitamin. The rest were various herbs and megadoses of vitamins and minerals.

## Ginkgo Biloba

*While some scientists thought there might be a slight improvement in dementia or in memory enhancement or other cognitive functions by taking* Ginkgo biloba *extracts or supplements, current research does not support that theory (more Pushmi-Pullyus). An article in the* Journal of the American Medical Association *reported that a six-year study in which people took 120 mg of* Ginkgo biloba *twice a day was not effective in reducing the overall incidence of Alzheimer's disease or other dementias. That said,* Ginkgo biloba *has been used in Chinese medicine for more than 1,000 years. The* Ginkgo biloba *tree has a life span of 2,000–4,000 years, and its presence on earth goes back 230 million years. Traditionally in Chinese medicine* Ginkgo *leaves or extracts from them have been used for heart and lung health, as anti-inflammatory and healing agents for tinnitus and asthma. Maybe Western medicine has not figured out the best way to harness the healing power of this ancient tree yet.*

*Do not take* Ginkgo biloba *if you are on a blood-thinning medicine like coumadin, since* Ginkgo *also increases blood thinning.*

I have to admit I got caught up in a scam, too. Years ago when I first went back to school to study exercise physiology and nutrition, I was talked into buying a "cleansing program" that would help me detoxify my body and lose weight. I spent about $100 and had to drink tasteless detoxifying rice-based shakes and not eat any "sugar" or white flour (honey and rice syrup were OK—I did not know then that they are virtually the same as "sugar"). I did lose weight, since I was hardly eating anything. I did not feel any less toxic, but I had not felt toxic in the first place. That company's founder has been fined by the FTC numerous times for making false health claims but is still in business today.

---

### Acetyl-l-carnitine

*Acetyl-l-carnitine has become a popular memory-enhancing supplement. Some studies suggested a beneficial effect on cognition and behavior, but larger studies have not supported those findings. Acetyl-l-carnitine has an antioxidant effect in the central nervous system and helps with cell and nerve health. More research needs to be done to see whether acetyl-l-carnitine supplementation has a positive effect on memory, cognition, or dementia.*

---

## The Salt of the Earth

Minerals are just as important as vitamins for a well-balanced, highly functioning brain and body. Some minerals we need in only tiny amounts: for instance, 40 mg a day of zinc and 45 mg a day of iron. Other minerals, such as sodium, we need more of: 2,300 mg a day. Getting minerals from food and your multi is the best way to maintain your body's mineral balance.

### Zinc and Iron

Both zinc and iron are essential in brain development and cognitive function. Dieting may deplete these minerals and affect reaction time, memory, and attention span.

**Healthy Foods High in Zinc**
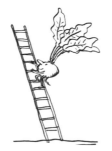
    Chickpeas
    Pecans
    Chicken breast
    Red beans
    Part-skim mozzarella

## Bacopa

*Bacopa monniera is a traditional Ayurvedic medicine that has been used for almost 3,000 years as a memory-enhancing, anti-inflammatory, analgesic, antipyretic, sedative, and antiepileptic agent. In India, Bacopa is also known as Brahmi, derived from the Hindu "Brahma, the mythical creator." At this time we do not know how Bacopa affects memory or cognition. A few small scientific studies done in humans examining the effects of Bacopa monniera on memory have had conflicting results. As with any herb or herbal tonic preparation, there can be interactions with certain medications. Caution is advised when taking an herb or tonic for which we have little evidence of its safety and efficacy.*

### Healthy Foods High in Iron
Lentils
Whole-grain breads
Turnip greens, collard greens
Turkey breast
Prunes

## Sodium

My grandmother used to have a small dish of kosher salt on her stove, and whenever I walked through her kitchen, I'd take a pinch and eat it. We are not born with a love for salt; it is a taste we acquire—except for me. My mom says I was born with a salt craving. She says that when I was little I'd reach up behind her in the kitchen and grab a handful of salted butter from the counter and eat it. I'd also shake salt into the palm of my hand and lick it off. It's a miracle I did not have high blood pressure by the time I was 12. I am better about my salt intake now. I don't eat handfuls of salted butter anymore.

Since the taste for salt is something we acquire from eating salty food, it will go away if you go low-salt or no salt for about two weeks. Your taste buds will adapt, and the foods you used to add salt to will now taste perfect without it. A heads-up to parents: If you steer your children away from high-sodium, high-fat foods, they will not develop a taste for them. There is absolutely no reason for little ones to be eating fast food, junk foods, or a lot of prepared foods.

**Salt Fact:** Sea salt, kosher salt, and regular salt are all the same thing. None is better or worse for you.

Nadine had come to see me because her physician told her she had borderline high blood pressure. I reviewed her diet and let her know that the current recommendation for sodium is 2,300 mg a day but warned her that most of us consume a lot more than that.

"Oh, I don't eat even half that," said Nadine.

When I pointed out that one teaspoon of table salt has 2,400 mg of sodium, she gulped. I continued to shock and amaze her by telling her that the baked stuffed shrimp she had at a restaurant the previous evening had 1,040 mg of sodium. Her favorite lunchtime Greek salad has 1,060 mg of sodium (it's the feta and salad dressing that do it). Estimates put the sodium intake of Americans at 4,000 mg a day or higher. After reading the May 2009 report by the Center for the Science in the Public Interest (CSPI) on the amount of sodium in chain restaurants, I'd say those estimates are ridiculously low. CSPI's investigators discovered that one meal could equal three days' worth of sodium! Here are a few of their results:

Red Lobster's Admirals' Feast with Caesar Salad, Creamy Lobster Topped Mashed Potato, Cheddar Bay Biscuit, and a Lemonade: 7,106 mg

Chili's Buffalo Chicken Fajitas (with tortillas and condiments) and a Dr Pepper: 6,916 mg

Olive Garden's Tour of Italy (lasagna) with a Breadstick, Garden Fresh Salad with House Dressing, and a Coca-Cola: 6,176 mg

These and other restaurant meals contain monstrous amounts of sodium. Your blood pressure will be skyrocketing before you even pay the check.

The recommendation for sodium is 2,300 mg a day. Most of us are eating a whole lot more than that.

Sodium, like potassium, iron, magnesium, and other minerals, is necessary for a healthy body. Sodium regulates fluid balance in cells and tissues, creates the electricity needed for neurons to transmit their electrochemical messages, and helps in the transport of certain molecules in and out of cells. We get the sodium we need from the foods we eat. However, in general we are eating a lot more sodium than we need.

When we eat too much sodium (dietary sodium), it can knock off the body's delicate balance of minerals and lead to problems in blood pressure and kidney function. Research suggests that dietary sodium contributes to the onset and prevalence of high blood pressure (also known as hypertension). Hypertension and dietary sodium are serious problems. In fact, in June 2006, the American Medical Association released a report urging the Food and Drug Administration to put warning labels on foods containing 480 mg or more per serving.

Eating a diet high in sodium increases your risk of developing high blood pressure.

### Sodium per Measure of Salt (sodium chloride)

*¼ teaspoon salt = 600 mg sodium*

*½ teaspoon salt = 1,200 mg sodium*

*¾ teaspoon salt = 1,800 mg sodium*

*1 teaspoon salt = 2,400 mg sodium*

*1 teaspoon baking soda = 1,000 mg sodium*

### Sodium and Your Brain

"I don't have hypertension. I don't feel nervous, and I am not stressed out," Joshua told me. He had not had his blood pressure checked in years. That's the problem with hypertension, also known as high blood pressure. You can't feel it. There are no symptoms, and you do not have to feel edgy or tense to have hypertension. The name is misleading. *Hypertension* sounds like a Wall Street executive on methamphetamines. The reality is that hypertension refers to the volume and pressure of blood in the arteries. Like a garden hose. How much water pressure you get depends on how much water is flowing through the hose. Turn the spigot on full blast and you can spray water all the way across the lawn. The volume of blood (which is mostly water) in the arteries depends on many factors, including sodium. The more sodium you consume, the more water is pulled into the arteries from surrounding tissues, the higher the pressure in the arteries, and the greater the strain on the cardiovascular system. Over time high blood pressure can damage the kidneys, arteries, and heart and increases the risk of stroke. High blood pressure is bad for the brain. Those little blood vessels in your head can only take so much excess pressure before they start to malfunction. High blood pressure is associated with cognitive dysfunction and de-mentia. Lowering the sodium in your diet and eating a lot of vegetables and fruits is a great way to help lower blood pressure. Vegetables and fruits are high in potassium, magnesium, and calcium, all of which help lower blood pressure.

*How many milligrams of sodium are in a breakfast consisting of 1 Dunkin' Donut corn muffin plus 1 Starbucks Grande Green Tea Frappuccino?*

> *a. 270 mg*
>
> *b. 1,160 mg*
>
> *c. 78 mg*

Answer: *b. 1,160 mg*

*That's more than half of a whole day's worth of sodium.*

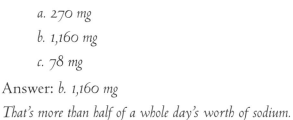

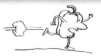

High blood pressure, aka hypertension, has no symptoms. Get your blood pressure checked regularly. Hypertension increases the risk of cardiovascular disease, stroke, dementia, and cognitive dysfunction.

You can find salt, which is a combination of two minerals, sodium and chloride, in just about every processed, boxed, or prepared food. Hiding the salt shaker is helpful but does not make as much of a difference as you think. More than 75 percent of the sodium we eat is in prepared, restaurant, frozen, and processed foods. Only 20 percent comes from the salt shaker. Sodium is hidden in foods like baked goods, sweets, breads, and beverages.

**It Doesn't Taste Salty!**
Foods do not have to taste salty to be loaded with sodium. Sodium is used as a flavor enhancer, for texture, and as a preservative. Additives like monosodium glutamate, disodium phosphate, garlic salt, and sodium benzoate can be a significant source of sodium in processed and frozen foods. You will also find sodium in products like baking soda and baking powder.

☞ Sodium has many important functions in the body.

☞ Sodium increases blood pressure.

☞ Limiting dietary sodium is a good idea.

☞ High blood pressure is tough on the brain.

☞ It is also bad for the cardiovascular system and kidneys.

☞ Sodium is hiding in unexpected places.

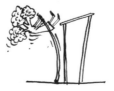

**Sodium in Popular Restaurant Food and Mall, Fast, and Frozen Foods**

| Food | Amount | Mg of Sodium |
|---|---|---|
| Chicken Giardino—entrée | 1 | 1,180 |
| Egg roll | 1 | 460 |
| Fast-food popcorn chicken | 6 oz | 1,050 |
| Pepperoni pizza | 1 slice, 4 oz | 790 |
| KFC fried chicken breast | 5½ oz | 1,120 |
| Burger King French toast sticks with syrup | 5 | 440 |
| Dunkin' Donuts corn muffin | 1 | 860 |
| McDonald's Chicken Selects Premium Breast Strips | 5 pieces | 1,550 |
| McDonald's Chocolate Triple Thick Shake | 32 oz | 510 |
| Starbucks Morning Sunrise Muffin | 1 | 550 |
| Starbucks Java Chip Frappuccino Light Blended Coffee—no whip | 1 | 350 |
| Swanson Hungry Man XXL Roasted Carved Turkey frozen dinner | 1 | 5,410 |
| V-8 Juice | 8 oz | 590 |
| Pepperidge Farm One-Step Stuffing chicken mix | ½ cup | 520 |
| Pepperidge Farm Homestyle French Toast, frozen | 1 slice | 200 |
| Krispy Kreme chocolate iced cake doughnut | 1 | 320 |
| Oscar Meyer turkey breast, fat free, smoked | 1 serving | 569 |
| Italian salad dressing | 2 tbs | 486 |
| Animal crackers | 1 box | 273 |
| White bread | 1 slice | 160 |
| Kellogg's Crispix cereal | 1 cup | 281 |

*Sources:* MF Jacobsen, JG Hurley, Center for Science in the Public Interest, Restaurant Confidential (New York: Workman, 2002); USDA National Nutrient Database for Standard Reference, Release 21, U.S. Department of Agriculture, Agricultural Research Service, 2009, www.ars.usda.gov/ ba/bhnrc/ndl; Dunkin' Donuts Web site, www.dunkindonuts.com/aboutus/nutrition/Product .aspx?Category=Bakery&id=DD-797; Pepperidge Farm Web site, www.pfwholegrains.com/ ProductDetail.aspx?prd_product_id=112032.

## What to Do

Whole fresh foods are your best options. Prepared foods like deli and restaurant food, processed foods, and soups are generally high in sodium. A processed food is any food that has been altered from its natural state. There are degrees. You can find low-sodium whole-grain breads (the flour has been made from the original whole grain, so technically it is processed). Read labels. Looks for the milligrams (mg) of sodium in foods. Ignore the percentages listed in the right-hand column.

## Going Low Sodium

| Food | Amount | Mg of Sodium |
|---|---|---|
| Regular peanut butter | 2 tbs | 147 |
| Unsalted peanut butter | 2 tbs | 5 |
| Regular tomato juice | 8 oz | 680 |
| Low-sodium tomato juice | 8 oz | 141 |
| Frozen broccoli, with salt, cooked | 1 cup | 478 |
| Frozen broccoli, no salt, cooked | 1 cup | 20 |
| Salami | 3 slices | 493 |
| Chicken breast, roasted, no skin | 3 oz | 64 |
| Pretzels, salted | 10 twists | 1,029 |
| Pretzels, unsalted | 10 twists | 173 |
| Cheddar cheese | 1 oz | 176 |
| Low-sodium cheddar cheese | 1 oz | 6 |
| Dunkin' Donuts corn muffin | 1 | 860 |
| Pepperidge Farm whole wheat English muffin | 1 | 210 |
| *Campbell's 25% Less Sodium Chicken Noodle Soup | ½ cup condensed, 1 cup prepared with water | 660 |
| Campbell's Healthy Request Chicken Noodle Soup | 1 cup | 480 |
| Campbell's Low-Sodium Chicken Noodle Soup | 1 cup | 140 |

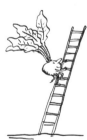

*Sources:* USDA National Nutrient Database for Standard Reference, Release 21, U.S. Department of Agriculture, Agricultural Research Service, 2009, www.ars.usda.gov/ba/bhnrc/ndl; Dunkin' Donuts Web site, www.dunkindonuts.com/aboutus/nutrition/Product.aspx?Category=Bakery&id=DD-797; Pepperidge Farm Web site, www.pfwholegrains.com/ProductDetail.aspx?prd_product_id=112032.
  *Note how confusing the various versions of a particular food can be, as shown by the various versions of Campbell's Chicken Noodle soup. You have to read and compare labels to know how much sodium you are getting.

See below for a list of foods high in sodium (these should be used sparingly). Some you should avoid (like luncheon meats and hot dogs), and some you can have with the idea that you can fit a certain amount of sodium in your day. For example, if you have soup for lunch from a restaurant, you can assume that will be a big chunk of your daily sodium.

## Foods High in Sodium
Just about all prepared sauces
Seasoning packets that come with rice, noodles, and salad dressings
Soy sauce (even the low-sodium version has about 500 mg per tablespoon)
Worcestershire sauce
Garlic, onion, and celery salt
Teriyaki sauce
Smoked sauces
Jarred gravies
Relish
Bottled or packet salad dressings
Marinades
Pasta sauces
Catsup (low-sodium or no-sodium versions are available)
Mustard
Luncheon meats—all!
Smoked or cured meats or fish—even smoked salmon
Sausages, hot dogs
Canned food (e.g., tuna, chicken, crab, clams)
Canned soups (you can get low-sodium or no-sodium soups in cans, but don't expect to find them in restaurants)
Tomato juice
Cheese (even the low-fat or no-fat cheeses tend to be high in sodium)
Pizza (tomato sauce is high in sodium)
Tomato: sauces, paste, canned (no-sodium-added versions available for all of these)
Pretzels, chips, crackers
Canned beans (the organic beans have less sodium than regular; dump the beans into a sieve and rinse well to reduce the added sodium)
Soy and other "meat" alternatives

## Low-Sodium or No-Sodium Flavor Boosters
Vinegars: e.g., balsamic, red wine, apple cider

---

### The Cheese Tray

*Cheese is loaded with artery-clogging saturated fat and cholesterol. It is also surprisingly high in sodium. One ounce of cheese is only about the size of your thumb. Low-fat (or nonfat), low-sodium cheeses are a better alternative. Remember to check the "nutrition facts" label. Low-fat cheeses can be high in sodium, and low-sodium cheeses can be high in fat.*

---

All herbs and spices, fresh or dried
Lemon
Hot spices if you like them: e.g., cayenne, chili pepper
Hot peppers
Mrs. Dash
Low-sodium salsas (the fruit salsas are usually a good choice)
Garlic, onions, shallots, leeks

Fresh vegetables and fruits are low in sodium and high in vitamins, minerals, antioxidants, and fiber that help lower blood pressure.

### What the Labels Mean

The following definitions are from an article that originally appeared in the September 1994 *FDA Consumer* and was revised (in September 1995) and reprinted online.

- **Sodium-free**: less than 5 milligrams (mg) per serving
- **Very low sodium**: 35 mg or less per serving or, if the serving is 30 grams (g) or less or 2 tablespoons or less, 35 mg or less per 50 g of the food
- **Low-sodium**: 140 mg or less per serving or, if the serving is 30 g or less or 2 tablespoons or less, 140 mg or less per 50 g of the food
    - **Salt-free**: sodium-free
    - **Unsalted, without added salt, no salt added:**
        —no salt added during processing, and
        —the food it resembles and for which it substitutes is
            normally processed with salt

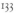

## Beware All-Natural

*We believe that "all natural" means healthy, safe, and good for you. We think of rolling hills, wildflowers, butterflies, and acres of farm-fresh vegetables. Let's get real. Dirt and dog poop are all natural, but you don't want to eat them. The truth is that all-natural foods can still be high in bad saturated fat, sugar, sodium, and calories and low in fiber, vitamins, minerals, phytochemicals, and antioxidants. All-natural herbs and supplements can contain all-natural insect parts and toxic substances. The FDA does not regulate these supplements, so you really have no idea what you are getting. If you are going to buy herbs, look for the U.S. Pharmacopeia's "USP Dietary Supplement Verified" seal, which indicates that the product has met certain manufacturing standards.*

**The Cheese Chart**

| Cheese: 1 oz | Calories | Saturated Fat (in grams) | Cholesterol (in mg) | Sodium (in mg) |
|---|---|---|---|---|
| Feta | 75 | 4.2 | 25 | 316 |
| Cheddar | 114 | 6 | 30 | 176 |
| Cream cheese | 99 | 6 | 31 | 84 |
| Brie | 95 | 5 | 28 | 178 |
| Gouda | 101 | 5 | 32 | 232 |
| American | 93 | 4 | 18 | 452 |
| Cheese Whiz Light, 2 tbs | 75 | 2 | 13 | 597 |
| Swiss | 107 | 5 | 26 | 54 |
| Mozzarella | 85 | 4 | 22 | 178 |
| Parmesan, grated, 1 tbs | 22 | 0.9 | 4.4 | 76 |

*Source:* Adapted from USDA Agricultural Research Service, Nutrient Data Laboratory, www.nal.usda.gov/fnic/cgi-bin/nut_search.pl.

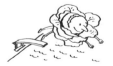

- Vitamins and minerals are essential for life.
- Getting your vitamins and minerals from food should always be your first choice.
- There are times when we need certain supplements.
- Taking a multivitamin and a 1,000-IU vitamin D supplement daily is a good idea.
- All the B vitamins play critical roles in brain function.
- All antioxidants, including vitamins C and E, are good for brain health.
- Minerals are necessary players for a healthy brain and body.
- Sodium is a must-have for neural communication, fluid balance, and cell transport.
- Most people eat too much sodium.
- The amount of sodium you eat has an impressive effect on blood pressure.
- High blood pressure is dangerous.
- Lowering the amount of sodium you eat every day helps lower blood pressure.
- Vegetables are especially helpful in lowering blood pressure due to their high content of vitamins and minerals, like potassium.

## CHAPTER FIVE

# Brainastics: Exercise

---— KEY POINTS ———

⇨ The brain can alter its capacity to accommodate new knowledge.

⇨ Physical exercise enhances brain function.

⇨ Regular exercise makes your brain and body physiologically younger.

⇨ Ab flab increases the risk of cognitive decline.

⇨ Being healthy and fit is more important than being thin.

⇨ Frequent cognitive activity is associated with reduced incidence of mild cognitive impairment and less rapid cognitive decline.

⇨ **People with greater social contacts and activities have a lowered risk of cognitive decline.**

⇨ **Sleep does a body good.**

——— NUTRITION PRESCRIPTION ———
*for* EXERCISE

⇨ **Exercise every day. Walk, dance, run, swim, kick-box, take an exercise class, swing your arms and wiggle your toes for a fit brain.**

## Brain Plasticity

THE FIRST TIME I heard the term *plastic brain*, I thought it was referring to Saran Plastic Wrap (this was before Press 'n' Seal). Then I learned that a plastic brain was one of those mini-miracles that happen in your body every day and that it has nothing to do with plastic wrap. Brain plasticity, also known as neuroplasticity, refers to the brain's ability to rewire neurons and connections and remap how the connections are made. As we grow and learn, the brain adapts its communication system to accommodate new information. Whether we are learning a skill like playing the piano, learning a new language, or playing a sport, the brain is constantly evolving and changing by creating new connections between neurons. This is especially evident in people who have suffered brain damage from strokes or traumatic brain injuries. When they learn how to walk and talk all over again, it is because the plasticity of the brain allows the creation of new neural networks to process new information.

As we get older, the brain is less plastic, less able to build new connections and acquire new knowledge. This decrease in plasticity affects learning, thinking, and memory. Once you hit your thirties, you start losing brain tissue and, as a result, cognitive function. But there are things you can do to hang on to those brain cells. Not only does exercise strengthen the heart, improve circulation, lower the risk of cancer, eat up excess body fat, improve mood, and reduce anxiety, it also helps slow the loss of brain tissue. In a study in the *Journal of Gerontology*, researchers took MRIs of people's brains and found a clear and specific

## A Confession

*All the stories in this book are true (though the names have been changed). I am a stickler for honesty—with one exception. When I get on a cardio machine at the gym and I have to enter my age and weight, I lie. I make myself younger and lighter. It's a white lie. I don't think it hurts anyone or affects national security.*

difference in brain matter between those who exercised regularly and those who did not. The exercisers had more white and gray matter than the nonexercisers (white and gray matter is made up of brain neurons). These results indicate that exercise is protective of and helps preserve brain matter.

The recommendations in *Get Smart* are based partly on what you can do to help maintain the brain's plasticity, reduce oxidative damage, and protect neurons and structures in the brain with healthy food and lifestyle. Regular aerobic (aka cardiovascular) exercise increases brain plasticity and reduces age-associated declines in cognitive function. In addition, scientists believe that regular exercise may repair or restore an aging brain, enhance cognitive performance, and improve memory.

The brain has this amazing ability to remodel and rewire its communication system among neurons so we can learn. Aerobic exercise supports and improves the brain's plasticity as well as protects brain tissue. People who exercise may have a delayed onset of Alzheimer's disease and other dementias.

## Smart Talk

Just saying "brain-derived neurotrophic factor" (BDNF) makes you feel smarter. BDNF is a compound found naturally in the brain that boosts synaptic activity (instant messaging in the brain) and supports the growth and survival of brain neurons. Another great effect of exercise is

## Rah Rah

*When I was in junior high school, we had to wear gym suits to gym class. They were ugly and stinky, and we all felt pretty foolish in them. Once I got to high school, I was thrilled that we did not have to take phys ed classes. I had no talent in team sports, but all my friends were pretty athletic. I tried cheerleading instead. It was the cool thing to do. Though I made the Junior Varsity cheerleading squad, I think it was more because the judges liked me than because I had any skill as a cheerleader. I mention this because there are some of us who are not cut out for team sports. However, kids of all ages are definitely cut out to run around and play and move their bodies. If your child is not interested in football or gymnastics, encourage him or her to find fun ways to be physically active. Join your kids in taking long walks, treasure hunts, Frisbee, badminton, jumping rope, swimming or dancing. If one of your children is a fashionista, do mall walks and scope out the sales.*

that it increases levels of BDNF. When you are engaged in heart-pumping activity, you are pumping up BDNF levels and thus pumping up your brain power, learning ability, and memory. Scientists do not know exactly why exercise has such a positive effect on both young and old brains. They speculate that it may have something to do with increased levels of BDNF and catecholamines and increased circulation (more blood to the brain). All we really need to know is that exercise improves cognitive function and boosts brain performance and memory.

Exercise helps preserve brain mass and brain function, thus reducing age-associated decline in cognitive function and memory.

☞     Brain plasticity is the brain's ability to acquire new knowledge and to learn.

☞ Brain-derived neurotrophic factor is necessary for healthy brain neurons.

☞ Exercise increases BDNF.

☞ Exercise increases circulation to the brain.

☞ Exercise appears to enhance the brain's ability to learn and stay young.

## Revive Your Old Jeans, uh . . . Genes, for the Ultimate Antiaging Solution

Both strength training and aerobic exercise turn on your inner fountain of youth! Strength training improves mental function and mood. Using weights or resistance machines or bands increases muscle mass, bone density, and balance and makes you feel good.

In an experiment published in the journal *PloS One*, scientists found that strength training changed the genetic profile of the participants to a more youthful form. Two times a week for six months, older participants engaged in a program that consisted of 3 sets of 10 repetitions for each of the following: leg press, chest press, leg extension, leg flexion, shoulder press, lat pull-down, seated row, calf raise, abdominal crunch, and back extension, and 1 set of 10 repetitions for arm flexion and arm extension. Researchers report that resistance training reversed some aspects of muscle aging on a cellular and genetic level.

Strength training reverses body aging all the way down to the genetic level.

British researchers studied 2,401 twins and found that regular exercise protects the aging of the protective caps on bundles in genes. Protecting these structures called telomeres protects the body against the aging process. People in their study who were sedentary had shorter (or aged) telomeres than their active counterparts. The study authors report that the most active subjects had telomeres the same length as people 10 years younger.

Thirty minutes of exercise daily not only improves overall health but also makes you younger from the inside out. Up to 10 years younger!

## These Boots Were Made for Walkin'

Is it crazy to think you can walk yourself younger? Crazy, maybe, but true. In 2004 the Nurses' Health Study found that physical activity, including walking, improved cognitive function in women between 70 and 81 years old. Physical activity made them about three years younger (physiologically) and was associated with a 20 percent lower risk of cognitive impairment. Talk about the fountain of youth! You can literally walk away the years, even in your eighties.

A study in the *Journal of the American Medical Association* discovered that exercise improved cognitive function in people who complained of memory problems with as little as three 50-minute sessions a week that consisted of walking or other aerobic exercise and strength training. Another study in the same journal reported that men who walk at least 2 miles a day are 1.8 times less likely than sedentary men to develop dementia over a follow-up period of six years. It is never too late to start an exercise program. But don't wait. Start moving your body today! The fountain of youth flows through your feet!

Cardiovascular exercise and strength training improve cognitive function at all ages.

## Too Tired to Exercise

We are overworked, overtired, and overstressed. We skip the workout in favor of watching Oprah talk about working out. We eat extra food to give us extra energy. Guzzle highly caffeinated "energy" drinks by the gallon. What else is a hard-working, exhausted person to do?

Contrary to common beliefs, exercise does not exhaust you. As a survival mechanism when challenged with increasing physical activity, the human body steps up to the plate and meets that challenge head-on. When you engage in cardiovascular exercise—for example, walking every day or using a stationary bike—your body meets that challenge by getting stronger and more powerful. Remember back in seventh-grade biology learning about little organelles in cells called mitochondria? (Or did you skip that class?) Mitochondria are the power plants in every cell in the body. They produce energy just like your local power company. The more you exercise aerobically, the more mitochondria the body makes to produce more energy. Regular cardiovascular exercise actually *gives* you energy. If you do not exercise on a regular basis, you'll be suffering from a power shortage, and that *will* make you tired.

**Physical Fitness Fact:** A study of more than two hundred children followed over a period of three years, through the ages 5 to 8 years, found that fewer than half of young boys and only one in eight girls meet the government guidelines for physical activity. The United Kingdom and the United States governments recommend that children take part in at least 60 minutes of moderate physical activity every day.

## TVs, Computers, and Games, Oh My

Kids who watch a lot of TV, more than two hours a day, and are not getting at least 60 minutes or more of daily physical activity are more likely to be fat. Overweight kids have a 70 percent chance of being overweight or obese adults. The chain continues, as being overweight or obese increases the risk of heart disease, diabetes, cancers, and cognitive decline at all ages. Limit how much time your kids and you spend in front of the TV and computer and playing video games (I say this as I have been sitting in front of my computer for hours now . . .). Exercise your brain by coming up with creative ways to spend your time physically and mentally.

Time spent watching too much TV or playing at the computer is often at the expense of physical activity and can lead to obesity, which increases the risk of a decline in health at all ages.

## The Ab Flab

TV viewing is associated with more ab flab. Ab flab is bad for many reasons, but in the context of *Get Smart*, ab flab in your forties increases the risk of dementia more than three decades later. A Kaiser Permanente study with more than 6,500 people found that people who were over-weight and had a large belly were 2.3 times more likely to develop dementia than were people with a normal weight and belly size. People who were both obese and had a large belly were 3.6 times more likely to develop dementia than those of normal weight and belly size. Those who were overweight or obese but did not have a large abdomen had an 80 percent increased risk of dementia. Ab flab increases oxidative stress and internal inflammation, which are bad for your brain and cardiovas-cular system.

The fat in our belly behaves differently than fat in other parts of the body. It causes more inflammation and oxidative stress and is a greater risk factor for disease than is fat in other parts of the body. The belly fat that hangs over our belt and deep fat that lies under our abdomi-nal muscles, called visceral fat, contribute to overall ab flab. In recent years scientists discovered that fat cells secrete hormone-like substances. Some of the substances have anti-inflammatory actions (adiponectins), and some increase inflammation (adipocytokines). The fat that builds up around the abdomen releases more inflammatory compounds than do other fat cells. In young and older people alike, abdominal obesity increases the risk of insulin resistance, diabetes, cardiovascular disease, hypertension, stroke, mortality, and cancer.

Ab flab in your forties or fifties increases your risk of dementia more than 30 years later.

## Measure for Measure

Pull out the tape measure and wrap it around your waist. The National Cholesterol Education Program says that if your waist is 40″ or more for men or 35″ or more for women, you've got ab flab worth worrying about. Those numbers seem generous to me. I would say that if your waist measure is even *approaching* those recommendations, you need to be extra careful.

## What You Can Do to Reduce Ab Flab

- Start walking, hopscotching, hula-hooping ASAP. The STRIDDE study, which came out in October 2006, found that people who exercised, including cardiovascular and abdominal work, lost visceral fat (located deep in the abdomen), subcutaneous fat (under the skin), and abdominal fat without making a change in how much they were eating. The more exercise the subjects did, the more ab flab was lost.
- Another important finding of the STRIDDE study is that relatively short periods of continued physical *inactivity* resulted in a sizable and significant increase in visceral abdominal fat. Couch potatoes beware. While you are just sitting there, the deep fat, the most dangerous kind, is accumulating in your gut.
- Cut out saturated fats. Scientific evidence suggests that reducing the amount of saturated fats, the kind found in butter, cheese, meat, and ice cream, may help reduce belly fat.
- Got seltzer? Binge drinking may be a contributor to belly fat. So cut down on or cut out your alcohol consumption.
- Smoking increases belly fat. Stop poisoning yourself and everyone around you. There is absolutely nothing good about smoking, unless you work for the tobacco companies.
- Chill out. Yale researchers found that non-overweight women who are vulnerable to the effects of stress are more likely to have excess abdominal fat.

☞   Watching TV is linked to more ab flab.

☞   Ab flab makes your brain flabby, too.

☞   A big belly in midlife increases your risk of dementia.

## Physical Activity Is a Luxury We Can All Afford

The need to move our bodies is embedded in our DNA, architectural design, and brains. Remember: exercise in whatever form you choose is not punishment. My friend Jesse had amyotrophic lateral sclerosis (ALS), also known as Lou Gehrig's disease. ALS is a progressive degenerative disease that affects the neurons in the brain and spinal cord that make muscles move. Eventually people with ALS cannot move their limbs, and the muscles associated with breathing and other life support functions fail. I used to go to Jesse's apartment a few times a week to give him massages, read to him, hang out, and help out. He could not move his arms or legs. Jesse would look at me and say, "If I could only get up and walk across the room, I'd be so happy." I learned a lot from Jesse during that time. I realized that I was fortunate to have the opportunity to make my body healthier with exercise. On days when I find myself muttering about having to work out, I think of Jesse, and my resistance vanishes.

## Smart Moves

You get smarter when you exercise. Girls exposed to more physical activity versus less physical activity in school showed better performance in math and reading. I wish I had known that. I would have done jumping jacks before math class.

A review article in the *Journal of Pediatrics* (in which the researchers examine the available studies in the medical literature on a particular subject and summarize the information) reports that physical exercise in school-age children has a positive influence on concentration, memory, classroom behavior, and intellectual performance. Unfortunately, physical education classes are often cut out of the school curriculum these days, so children need to run, play, and jump after school and on the weekends.

Bernie, an 84-year-old patient of mine, has heart disease. He told me that even though he forced himself to come to our three-month cardiac rehab program, which meant exercising three times a week, he still hated exercise.

"I have no intention of continuing exercise now that the program is over," he said.

I offered many suggestions, but he shot them all down. Not willing to give up, I made a final try. "Do you dance, Bernie?"

He smiled, smoothed his hands on his seersucker pants, and replied, "I used to cut quite a rug back in the day. Tango, you know."

I encouraged him to find some tango classes or nearby clubs where he and his wife could go dancing. There is a whole tango subculture in New York City that includes lessons, competitions, clubs, and performances. Exercise does not have to be a stationary bike or boot camp class. It can be anything you enjoy doing. Try dance, Pilates, spinning, or sculpting class. Join a softball, tennis, or paddleball team. Start a neighborhood walking program.

☞ Physical activity makes both kids and adults smarter.

☞ Learning to tango may help you live longer.

## What to Do

- If you have been sedentary, see your doctor before beginning a new exercise program.
- Walking is always a good way to start. It's free, and you already know how to do it. All you need are a good pair of walking shoes and weather-appropriate clothing.
- Join a gym or fitness center that is convenient to where you work or live.
- Before you join a gym, check it out at the times you are most likely to work out. See whether you like the vibe, lighting, layout, and smell (sounds weird, but it can make a difference in motivation).
- Get qualified instruction.
- See what your Parks and Recreation Department or continuing education programs have to offer.
- Try something new, like a salsa or hip-hop dance class.
- Do not feel intimidated because a class or fitness machine is new to you. No one is looking at you. All the other people there are concerned with themselves.
- Go with a friend.
- Do not overdo it at the beginning.
- Be patient.

- Check with your health insurance company. Sometimes you can get discounts to fitness centers or classes.

## A Weighty Discussion

When one talks about exercise, it is inevitable that the discussion veers to weight loss. *Get Smart* is not about getting skinny. It is about creating healthy lifestyle behaviors that help promote optimal brain function and total body health. If you are overweight or obese, your risks of chronic disease and cognitive decline are significantly increased. More than 12.5 million children ages 2 to 19 years were overweight in 2004, and 32.2 percent of adults (more than 66 million) were obese. And it is not getting better. Eating a healthy diet and being physically active daily will make a big difference in overall health. By making a few simple changes every day, you can alter your brain and heart health and eventually your weight. Science has finally caught up with the notion that being healthy does not mean being skinny and vice versa. Being either overweight or underweight may increase the risk of developing dementia.

Just because someone is thin does not mean that he or she is healthy. Robert, a designer-clothing-store executive, was at a lean healthy weight when at 38 he suffered a mild heart attack. By his own admission he had been eating a diet high in artery-clogging saturated fat (pepperoni pizza for lunch—"But I'm Italian," he moaned). He did not work out and told me he figured walking around New York City was enough exercise for him. Robert thought that since he was thin he could eat anything he wanted. A common misconception. No matter what your weight is, eating a diet of predominantly unhealthy foods or not exercising (or both) can make you sick. If your genes are leaning in the direction of disease or dementia, then lifestyle can either magnify or minimize that potential.

Make healthy choices every day for a fit brain and body. If you are exercising and eating well and happen to be a few pounds overweight, that is better than being thin, eating badly, and sitting on your rump.

☞    Being overweight or obese increases the risk of developing many chronic diseases, including cognitive decline.

☞    Everyone needs to eat healthy foods and exercise regardless of his or her weight.

## What to Do

- Dump cheese on Monday, butter on Tuesday, and red meat on Thursday.
- Walk every day.
- Drink more water or seltzer.
- At mealtime, make sure vegetables take up half your plate. Healthy protein like chicken, soy, or beans should take up a quarter of your plate, and whole grains like whole-wheat pasta or brown rice should take up the other quarter.

## Mental Muscle

We know that watching a lot of TV can make you fat—or at least contribute to fatness. But now studies are showing that watching TV zaps your brain. In a study of more than 5,000 people in China, scientists found that people who played games and read in their leisure time had a reduced risk of cognitive impairment. More time spent watching TV was associated with an increased risk of cognitive impairment. There are many ways people can flex their brain muscles. Intellectual stimulation is another way to keep the brain sharp throughout the life span.

A study published in the journal *Neurology* that included 700 older people and spanned five years found that cognitively active people were less likely to develop Alzheimer's disease than were cognitively inactive people. Frequent cognitive activity was also associated with reduced incidence of mild cognitive impairment and less rapid decline in cognitive function. You can start revving your brain now by thinking of all the things you can think about!

### Challenge Your Brain

- Learn a new language.
- Take a class in anything that interests you.
- Learn a new skill such as painting, crocheting, woodworking, or playing a musical instrument.
- Brush your teeth with your other hand (if you normally brush with the right hand, use the left).
- Use utensils with your nondominant hand.
- Get dressed with your eyes closed.
- Drive a totally different route to the store or to work.
- Take a trip to a new place, even if it is only a few miles away.
- Go to a museum.
- See a play.
- Read a new book often.
- Rearrange your drawers.
- Memorize the lyrics to a new song.
- Do brain teasers such as word games.
- Play Scrabble, chess, and cards.
- Break any routine and do something new (this does not include watching a new TV show).
- Take a new kind of exercise or dance class.

☞ Watching more than two hours of TV a day can turn you and your children into the Zombie Family.

☞ Challenging the brain with new tasks and information such as reading, playing games, or learning new skills improves brain function.

## What's the Story, Morning Glory? What's the Tale, Nightingale?

Socializing is another important way you can decrease your risk of cognitive decline. Ongoing research is finding that people with greater social contacts and activities have a lowered risk of cognitive decline and dementia and experience delays in memory loss. Join a book club, take a class, visit friends and family, get involved with your community groups, join a church, take part in your local theater, or sing in a chorus.

## You Snooze, You Win

Getting too little sleep (less than five hours a night) or too much sleep (eight to nine hours) increases the risk of obesity. It seems like there is an epidemic of sleep disorders out there. The National Sleep Foundation 2008 report found that 65 percent of people surveyed reported sleep problems. Lack of sleep has been linked to cardiovascular disease, high blood pressure, decreased learning ability, and slower thinking process-es. A good night's rest is imperative for a well-functioning brain. Here's how to do it.

### Six Ways to Get Better Sleep

1. Stick to a sleep schedule: go to bed and get up at the same time every day. Your body will adapt to the schedule, making the best of its sleep time.
2. Avoid caffeine: caffeine can stay in your system as long as eight hours. Do not drink caffeinated beverages later in the day.
3. Skip the nightcap: alcohol may make you sleepy, but it wakes you up in the middle of the night and makes it difficult to get back to sleep. Alcohol robs you of your deep and REM sleep.
4. Eat light at night: big late-night meals can exacerbate gastric reflux, especially if you lie down within two hours after eating. They can also make you physically uncomfortable and less likely to get a good night's sleep.
5. Unwind before bed: don't jump into bed all revved from the day. Give yourself time to unwind and chill out before hitting the sack. Read a book, page through a magazine, take a hot bath or shower.
6. Sleeping quarters: keep your sleep environment dark and cool. Remove things like ticking clocks or computers that may distract you from sleep.

- **Physical exercise can help the brain form new neural pathways to accommodate learning and new skills.**

- **Physical exercise keeps the brain young and healthy by improving circulation and increasing brain-derived neurotrophic factor.**

- **Mental exercises also help keep the brain young and improve cognitive function as we age.**

- **Both mental exercise and physical exercise need to be kept up at all ages.**

- **Socializing helps reduce the risk of dementia and improves memory.**

- **A good night's sleep can work wonders.**

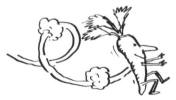

# CHAPTER SIX

# Cheers to Your Health! Alcohol, Caffeine, and the Brain

---

### KEY POINTS

---

⇨ Alcohol is toxic to the body.

⇨ Alcohol consumption causes approximately 100,000 deaths annually in the United States.

⇨ Alcohol may be protective against dementia.

⇨ It's difficult to drink "moderately."

⇨ **If you do not now drink alcohol, don't start.**

⇨ **Caffeine is a stimulant.**

⇨ **Caffeine is OK to consume in reasonable amounts and may improve cognitive function.**

## A Slippery Slope

ALCOHOL MAKES YOU DRUNK and causes wicked hangovers and many regrets. It is addictive. Chronic alcohol consumption can cause cirrhosis of the liver and progressive neurodegenerative disease (brain rot). Alcohol is high in calories. Per gram it has almost twice as many calories as protein or carbohydrates. In addition, prolonged or excessive alcohol consumption has been associated with an increased risk of dementia. An article in the *Journal of the American College of Cardiology* sums up the effects of drinking alcohol nicely:

> Excessive alcohol intake increases the risks of motor vehicle accidents, stroke, cardiomyopathy, cardiac dysrhythmia, sudden cardiac arrest, suicide, cancer (most notably of the breast and gastrointestinal tract), cirrhosis, fetal alcohol syndrome, sleep apnea, and all-cause mortality.

Thus it is natural for me to want to tell you not to drink alcohol at all. However, the scientific Pushmi-Pullyus have trotted into this arena, too. There's an upside to drinking alcohol, especially wine.

Alcohol contains antioxidants and other compounds, such as resveratrol, that may be cardio-protective as well as neuro-protective. Research studies that have examined the relationship between alcohol consumption and dementia suggest that there might be an association between small to moderate amounts of alcohol and a reduced risk of dementia. For example:

- The Nurses' Health Study found that in women, up to one drink per day does not impair cognitive function and may actually decrease the risk of cognitive decline.

- In people with mild cognitive impairment, up to one drink per day of wine or other alcohol may decrease the rate of progression to dementia.
- A study with a 34-year follow-up (a really long time in science) found that in women wine was protective against dementia but that beer and spirits may increase the risk of dementia.
- The Cardiovascular Health Study reported that compared with nondrinkers people who drank one to six drinks weekly had a lower risk of incident dementia among older adults.

## To Drink or Not to Drink

Chris, a friend of mine, is 47 years old; he is in good physical shape but has low HDL (good) cholesterol. He asked me whether he should start drinking red wine every night to try to raise his HDL levels. He heard that red wine would raise his HDLs and be good for his heart. "No," I said. "Alcohol adds unnecessary calories and makes it easy to gain weight. You'd be better off increasing foods high in niacin, a B vitamin that raises HDLs." Being a musician who plays mostly in bars, he went the red wine route. Three months later, after having red wine every night, his HDLs were no better and he'd started putting on weight. I do not like to say "I told you so." Instead I said, "Chris, I do not like to say I told you so but, well . . . I did."

Do not start drinking alcohol if you do not drink now. If you do drink alcohol, chances are you need to lower your consumption. It is a slippery slope for folks to have only one or two small drinks at a time. Not many can limit themselves to that. In addition, alcohol may interact with certain medications and increase the risk of liver damage. If you are on any medications, consult with your physician about drinking alcohol.

## Cup o' Joe

My mother's mantra was "Don't talk to me until I've had my first cup of coffee." She needed that caffeine boost before she could even think of dealing with children. As early as Starbucks and diners are open in

**Caffeine Content in Coffee and Tea**

| Coffee or Tea | Caffeine (in mg) |
| --- | --- |
| 8 oz cup brewed coffee | 80–100 |
| 16 oz Starbucks Frappuccino | 110 |
| 16 oz Starbucks coffee of the week | 330 |
| 1 oz espresso | 75 |
| 16 oz Starbucks Chai Tea Latte | 100 |
| 8 oz brewed black tea | 47 |
| 8 oz brewed green tea | 20 |

New York City (some are open all night), lines form as people on their way to work grab their morning cup o' Joe before they can even think of starting their workday. Caffeine is the most widely consumed over-the-counter drug in the world. We keep waiting for someone to tell us caffeine is bad for our health, but so far there is no research to support that notion for normal caffeine consumption. Caffeine is addictive, as you know if you are a caffeine drinker and tried to go off the stuff. You may have gotten a bad headache or nausea as you went through withdrawal. The current boom in energy drinks has become a $5.7 billion industry as kids and adults chug these highly caffeinated beverages that also contain other stimulants. I am not a fan of these drinks, since they go way over the top. If you need that much artificial voltage to get through the day, then you probably are burning the candle at both ends and need to get more sleep and eat better. But I digress. Caffeine and the brain.

Caffeine, a central nervous system stimulant, which we usually consume in coffee, tea, sodas, and, now, energy drinks, has a direct biochemical effect on the brain. As we discussed Chapter 2, neurotransmitters can have excitatory or calming effects on the brain. Caffeine blocks a naturally occurring brain substance called adenosine, which has a calming influence in the brain. Thus the balance between excitatory and calming neurotransmitters is thrown to the excitatory side and you feel alert, awake, and focused. Too much caffeine takes you over the edge, and you get jittery, cranky, and shaky. Caffeine itself is not an energy source. It changes brain chemistry to produce more excitatory chemicals in the body. So if you are low on energy and keep drinking

**Caffeine and Guarana Content in Energy Drinks and Sodas**

| Drink | Amount | Caffeine (in mg) | Guarana (in mg) |
|---|---|---|---|
| Rockstar | 1 bottle | 160 | 50 |
| Amp Energy Overdrive | 1 can | 160 | 248 |
| Sugarfree Red Bull | 8 oz | 80 | 0 |
| Diet Pepsi Max | 8 oz | 46 | 0 |
| Jolt | 23.5 oz | 280 | 56 |
| Sobe Adrenaline Rush | 8 oz | 78 | 0 |
| Glaceau Vitamin Water Energy Citrus | 8 oz | 50 | 25 |

Sources: Product Web site or product label.

caffeine, eventually you will crash, since your body has only so much energy without being refueled with proper food and sleep.

In terms of cognitive function, caffeine does improve alertness, vigilance, and other mental functions. On the extreme side, a study done in the military found that high doses of caffeine helped sleep-deprived special forces team members maintain both vigilance and physical performance during sustained operations. On a more normal level, a study in France called the Three City Study found that in a group of more than 7,000 people caffeine consumption was associated with reduced cognitive decline and better memory in women without dementia, especially at higher ages. And another study found that lifetime and current exposure to caffeine was linked with better cognitive performance among women, especially those over 80 years old. No one yet knows why the positive cognitive effects of caffeine are seen more in women than in men. The stimulatory effects, though, are similar in both men and women.

If you are feeling foggy, a cup of caffeine in the form of coffee and, to a lesser extent, tea may give you the temporary clarity you need. I'd steer clear of energy drinks, since they contain not only caffeine but other central nervous system stimulants such as guarana. Besides, they are expensive. It is important to remember that caffeine can interfere with sleep, increase anxiety, and contribute to the jitters.

- Do not start drinking alcohol if you do not drink now.
- If you do drink, limit your consumption.
- If you are taking medication, consult your physician about interactions with alcohol.
- Caffeine is a central nervous system stimulant.
- Caffeine affects neurotransmitters in the brain.
- Caffeine increases mental alertness, vigilance, physical performance, and memory.
- Lifetime consumption of caffeine may reduce cognitive decline.
- Too much caffeine is not a good thing.

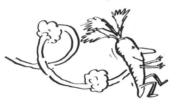

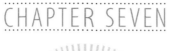

## CHAPTER SEVEN

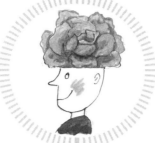

# Tips for Success

IN THIS WORLD OF fast, cheap, supersized food, it can be a challenge to find healthy foods and make healthy choices all the time. It is definitely doable and gets easier once you learn to navigate food courts, eating out, social occasions, traveling, and work. Here are some tips to make your journey to a healthier brain and body easier.

### Be Specific. Set goals and objectives.

Setting realistic goals and objectives is a very important part of any lifestyle change. For example, trying to lose 15 pounds by the end of the month is unrealistic. Reasonable goals might include learning to cook healthy foods, losing one to two pounds a week, beginning an exercise program, or seeing a registered dietitian. Objectives may include not snacking after dinner, eating breakfast every day, eating less saturated fat, walking 30 minutes a day, or including vegetables at lunch and dinner.

### Personalize your plan.

How are you going to reach those goals? Your plan has to be specific to your daily life. Be precise about how you are going to achieve your goals. How, for example, can you make your lunch healthier? Where do you usually eat lunch? Is it reasonable to think you will bring your lunch to work? If not, where will you eat and what will you choose for lunch?

## Plan ahead.

Planning ahead is the key to changing your habits. Write a meal-by-meal plan to help you get organized. Take into account where you live and work and what is realistic in terms of your daily life.

## Be prepared.

Stock your pantry with healthy foods such as legumes (beans), whole grains, vegetables, fruits, non-fat dairy products, nuts, and seeds. Then if you have a "snack attack," you can choose from a variety of lower-calorie, healthier foods. Plus, you will have all the ingredients you need to prepare your meals.

## Life's Little Potholes

It is easy to get sucked into our fast and cheap food culture. Here are some potholes you will come across in your quest for a healthier brain and body and ways to avoid them.

### Sneaking Weight

When autumn comes, the days get shorter and cooler. You rummage through your closet and select your favorite pair of pants from last year. You step into them and notice that they are harder to get over your thighs than you remember and the button at the waist is about to pop. Oh, you think, they must have shrunk in the wash. I could not have gained weight. Surprise! A few pounds probably did sneak past your radar. If you eat 100 calories a day more than your body needs, you can put on 10 pounds in a year. Maybe you do not sit down and eat a half a gallon of ice cream in a sitting, but little things add up.

- 4 tablespoons of ice cream = 135 calories, 4.5 grams saturated fat
- 1 ounce of cheese (about the size of the tip of your thumb) = 114 calories, 6 grams saturated fat
- 1 Snickers bar = 280 calories, 5 grams saturated fat
- 3 slices of salami = 105 calories, 3.3 grams saturated fat, 493 mg sodium (wow)

## Pretzels

I love mall pretzels. My friend Pat gets the no-fat no-salt mall pretzels. But those just don't cut the mustard with me. I allow myself a mall pretzel a few times a year. Those giant street and mall pretzels are high in calories and sodium. One original Pretzel Time pretzel has 390 calories and 220 mg of sodium. It tastes good but does not even fill you up. The white flour with which these pretzels are made will leave you hungry sooner than later. Most snack bag pretzels are made with refined flour. Get the whole-wheat no-salt pretzels. Have them with hummus or other healthy dip. Beware: these are devious little snacks. Before you know it, the whole bag is gone. Take out a handful as your portion and put the rest away.

## Sat Fat Foods

If you have a barbeque coming up and have an incurable desire for Uncle Bob's famous BBQ ribs, then go right ahead. My suggestion is to limit all foods high in saturated fat to twice a month, so plan ahead for occasions when you might want to indulge. Cheese feels like a very different food than ice cream, which feels different than butter, which feels different than steak, which feels a lot different than cake. But all these foods are high in bad saturated fat. This means that if you have Uncle Bob's ribs this weekend you have one other time this month to have a sat fat food like ice cream or cheese. Watch your portions too. Stick to 3–4 oz of high fat proteins, ½ cup of real ice cream and 2–3 oz of full fat cheese.

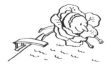

## Energy, Granola, Health, and Diet Bars

Many of these are glorified candy bars. All bars are not created equal. If you must grab a snack bar, choose the whole-grain bars that have fewer than 200 calories, less than 1 gram of saturated fat, and at least 2 grams or more of fiber (obviously no trans fats).

## Muffins

When I first moved to New York, I'd go across the street to a diner and have a bran muffin with butter and a cup of coffee for breakfast. I thought a bran muffin was a healthy choice. Besides the fact that the muffins were ginormous, they were probably a good 600 calories, crammed with saturated fat from the butter with which they were made and the butter I put on them. No wonder I started becoming a chunkette. You can make healthy muffins at home, but whole-grain, low-sat-fat, no-trans-fat, reasonably sized muffins are tough to find in stores or restaurants.

## Candy Bars

Need I say anything about candy? Of course I will. Betsy had just started going back to school and was working several jobs. She said she was always tired. She did not drink coffee, so to boost her energy she started buying candy bars. She did get an energy boost from the sugar, but it was followed by a resounding crash, and she had trouble staying awake in class. What Betsy really needed was to get more sleep and eat better foods that would fuel her body properly. Candy tastes really good. That's all that is good about it. Eating candy regularly is an excellent way to gain weight, waste money, lose brain power, and contribute to the risk of chronic diseases. Two small chocolate truffles are 220 calories.

## Tips for Brain-Healthy Eating at Work

Eating at work can become a real obstacle course. Colleagues order pizza. Some "thoughtful" secretary brings in a huge box of doughnuts in the morning. Your boss's birthday celebration includes a to-die-for chocolate mousse cake. The best thing you can do is "just say no." These "special occasions" happen almost daily. If you eat breakfast and lunch, you will be less tempted to dive into the office candy jar or grab a doughnut as you walk by the box.

## What to Do

- Eat breakfast! Go for whole-grain cereals like shredded wheat and oatmeal; multigrain waffles; nonfat yogurt with 2 tablespoons of granola mixed in; whole-wheat bagel with low-fat or tofu cream cheese; egg white omelet with spinach and onions on a slice of whole-wheat bread.
- Bring your lunch! Plan ahead for the week when you go to the grocery store. Get into the habit of packing your lunch the night before. Bring peanut butter and jelly on whole-grain bread, soy cheese, 3 ounces of tuna with low-fat mayo and lettuce and tomato, a drizzle of balsamic vinegar on whole-wheat bread, hummus with cucumber slices and chopped tomato and onions in a whole-wheat pita. Got a microwave at work? Try bringing pasta with marinara sauce and vegetables or leftover steamed vegetables with brown rice with a dash of low-sodium soy sauce.
- If packing a lunch is impossible, explore the neighborhood around your office. Find stores and restaurants that have healthy food choices.
- Watch out for the salad bar! Macaroni salad, tuna salad, coleslaw, and even carrot salad are usually swimming in mayonnaise! Stick with the fresh vegetables, mixed greens, chickpeas and kidney beans, and low-fat salad dressing or oil and vinegar.
- Do not be swayed by co-workers who are indulging in high-fat, unhealthy meals and snacks. Remember, your health is your number one priority.
- Keep healthy snacks handy—baby carrots, strips of red, yellow, and orange peppers, zucchini sticks, cherry tomatoes, cut-up fresh fruit, sesame whole-wheat pretzels, rice cakes.
- For that late-in-the-day sweet craving have a skim-milk hot chocolate (no whip). You get the chocolately taste with a dose of calcium and vitamin D.

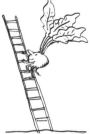

- If you order out, order pizza with no cheese (or low-fat cheese) and lots of vegetables. Try 3 ounces grilled chicken on a bed of mixed greens with low-fat dressing on the side, a grilled vegetable wrap, a spinach and black bean burrito (some restaurants even have low-fat sour cream or soy sour cream), baba ganoush on whole-wheat pita with chopped cucumbers, tomatoes, and onions.
- For afternoon snacks go for a nonfat yogurt, fresh fruit, mini rice cakes with a schmeer of low-fat cottage cheese, a handful of roasted soy nuts or oat bran pretzel nuggets, 2 whole-wheat graham crackers with a smudge of peanut butter.
- As tempting as office sweets may be, do not nibble on them. They may taste good but are packed with unnecessary and non-nutritive calories.
- Drink plenty of water—keep a bottle on your desk and sip all day.
- Take a movement break instead of a "coffee break." Walk around the block or up and down some stairs to get your energy moving.

## Shopping Lists

For fast, easy meals and snacks, stock your pantry and refrigerator with healthy foods. You can add or subtract choices depending on your preferences.

Carbohydrate Shopping List

Remember to choose whole grains.

Whole-grain bread
Whole-wheat pasta
Whole-wheat couscous (this cooks up in no time)
Whole-wheat pitas
Oatmeal
Oat bran
100 percent whole-grain ready-to-eat cereals
Whole-grain crackers, pretzels (no salt)
Whole-grain tortillas, pita chips

Corn tortillas
Farro pasta (for a change)
Quinoa
Brown and wild rices
Soy crisps, rice cakes
Baked chips
Whole-grain crackers (check the label to be sure they do not
contain partially hydrogenated oils)
Whole-grain pancake mix
Frozen, trans-free, whole-grain waffles
Whole-grain English muffins
Whole-wheat bagels (mini or regular)
No-fat popped corn

## Protein and Fat Shopping List

Avoid saturated and trans fats and foods high in cholesterol.

White-meat skinless chicken, turkey (organic if you can find/
afford it)
Egg whites or Egg Beaters
Fish: salmon, sole, tilapia, orange roughy, sardines, etc.
Soy foods: tofu, edamame, yuba, soy milk, soy nuts, soy cheese
Legumes: kidney beans, chickpeas, black-eyed peas, lentils, split
peas, etc. (Hint: rinse beans out of the can to reduce the sodium.
Organic beans have less added sodium.)
Hummus (all flavors)
Fat-free organic milk, cheese, yogurt, cottage cheese, sour cream
Low-fat cream cheese (the fat free is not all that tasty)
Fat-free half and half
Fat-free frozen yogurt, ice cream
Olive, canola (expeller pressed, organic), sesame, peanut, walnut oils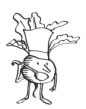
Peanut, almond, cashew butters ("natural")
Nuts (roasted, unsalted)
Seeds: pumpkin, sunflower, flax (ground)
Vegetarian chili (canned, low sodium)
Frozen soy or vegetarian soy nuggets, meatballs, grillers, sausages,

and bacon. Note: these can be high in sodium.
Frozen veggie burgers
Dr. Praeger's veggie burgers, spinach pancakes, and other similar products (frozen)

## Miscellaneous Shopping List

Low-sodium fat-free soups
Low-sodium low-fat healthy frozen entrees
Low-sodium tomato sauce
Low-sodium salsa and bean dips
No-added-sodium canned organic diced tomatoes
Tomato paste
70 percent or more cocoa, dark chocolate
All-fruit fruit pops

## Condiments Shopping List

Light or low-fat mayo
Mustard
Vinegars: balsamic, cider, wine, raspberry, etc.
Mrs. Dash
Fresh and dried herbs and spices (all are good)
Ketchup: low sodium or no salt added
Tahini (sesame paste—good for salad dressings, to drizzle on vegetables)

## Fruits and Vegetables Shopping List

Buy any and all you like and even some you don't. Definitely try vegetables and fruits you have not tried before.

Fresh or frozen (no salt or sauce added to the package)
Canned—no sodium
Dried figs
Prunes
Dried cranberries, raisins, for salads, muffins, and pilafs

## CHAPTER EIGHT

# Putting It Together, Bit by Bit

Now THAT YOU HAVE the basic prescription for a healthy brain, it's time to take action. I've created a two-week Kick Start Plan to help you get on the right track. You can pick and choose among the meal suggestions and add other healthy ingredients if you like. The reason the Kick Start Plan is not written in stone with calorie counts and a day-by-day meal plan is to help you learn to make your own healthy-brain choices. You can insert foods you like and skip the ones you don't. You can modify foods according to your budget and what is available.

This plan can work for you. Lisa was a student in a series of nutrition classes I teach at the local YMCA. A lot of what I teach is included in this book. Lisa came to class regularly, asked a few questions, but seemed pretty quiet most of the time. In the last class I asked the students to let me know what they liked about the class, what they learned, and what they might have liked to learn more about. Lisa spoke up and said, "I have lost 10 pounds since I started this class just by making healthier choices. I have not been 'dieting' or starving myself. I am trying to get my kids and husband on track too." Six months later I was out running and a car went by; the driver beeped and pulled over. It was Lisa. "I am so happy I ran into you," she said (technically I was the one who was running). "Since the end of class I have lost 25 pounds and my husband has lost 20 pounds."

"Lisa, how did you do it?" I asked.

"I am eating healthy foods, reading labels, watching my portions, and not going back for seconds. I feel so much better than I did at this time last year."

As I said in the beginning, this is not a diet book, but when you make healthy choices more often than not, watch your portion sizes, and start exercising, you may just lose those pesky extra pounds at the same time you are getting a healthier brain and body.

## Two-Week Kick Start Plan

The Kick Start Plan is vegetarian. It will help you break the cycle of eating meat, cheese, and full-fat dairy products and will drastically reduce your intake of saturated (bad) fat, cholesterol, and calories. The only dairy foods should be low-fat or nonfat and organic if you can find it and can afford it. You do not have to become a vegetarian forever. Just for two weeks. You can also substitute any of the vegetarian recipes in this book and use them during the Two-Week Kick Start Plan. This is a loose guide. You are in control of your choices and portions.

There is a lot of room for variation to accommodate your food preferences and budget. The Kick Start Plan is designed using foods that are easy to find or prepare. The measures are general estimates. It is good for you to learn to monitor your own portion sizes and feelings of satiety (comfortably full but not stuffed). Start by putting less on your plate than you think you want.

## Here are your Get Smart Nutrition Prescription Guidelines for the Kick Start Plan:

- Avoid foods with saturated fats and cholesterol.
- Choose protein with every meal—soy, nuts, low-fat or nonfat dairy, legumes.

- Have vegetables with at least two meals a day, three if you can swing it.
- The majority of your grains should be whole grains, though white pasta at the Italian restaurant or white rice at the Indian restaurant may be unavoidable.
- Have fruit one to two times a day
- Drink beverages with each meal and snack.

These are suggestions. You can mix and match. If you do not like peanut butter, that's fine. Try the hummus on whole-wheat pita instead. You can also try sunflower butter if you have a peanut allergy.

More guidelines:

- Never get overhungry or skip meals.
- Eat until you are satisfied but not stuffed.
- Monitor your portion sizes. Do not overdo it. For example, a serving of pasta is about 1–1½ cups, not the 3 cups we usually see at restaurants.
- There are several options for each meal and snack. Feel free to have a "breakfast" meal at lunch or vice versa.
- You can always add more vegetables.
- Drink plenty of fluids.
- Be adventurous. Try new foods.
- Eat slowly.
- Improvise with healthy ingredients.
- All herbs and spices are good—except salt.
- When eating out, be sure to ask your server how the food is prepared and then tell him or her how *you* want it prepared. No butter, cream, salt, or cheese.

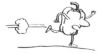

# *Kick Start Plan Options*

## BREAKFAST

(1) 2 organic egg white omelet (or scrambled) with
½ cup or more cooked spinach, broccoli, mushrooms, peppers, onions
(any vegetables you like), cooked in nonstick pan
1–2 tablespoons of low-sodium salsa or a dab of ketchup (optional)
Whole-wheat toast
1 tangerine

(2) 1 cup Kashi GO LEAN, shredded wheat, Total, All-Bran, or other 100
percent whole-grain cold ready-to-eat cereal (nothing frosted, please)
½–¾ cup organic nonfat milk or soy, rice, or almond milk
2 tablespoons ground flaxseeds
½ teaspoon of sugar or honey to taste (optional)
Optional: ½ cup berries or ½ banana

(3) ½ cup dry oatmeal (not the packets), cooked with water, no salt
2 teaspoons chopped almonds or walnuts
2 teaspoons flaxseed oil (add after oatmeal is cooked)
½ cup nonfat milk or soy, rice, or almond milk
½ teaspoon of sugar or honey to taste (optional)
1 tablespoon raisins or dried cranberries
Pinch of cinnamon

(4) Whole-wheat English muffin, brushed with 1 teaspoon canola oil
2 slices fat-free or low-fat cheese, or soy cheese, put under broiler until
cheese starts to melt (keep an eye on it)
Sliced tomato on top of melted cheese
¼ slice of cantaloupe or honeydew melon

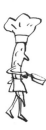

(5) 2 slices whole-wheat or 100 percent whole-grain bread, toasted
2 tablespoons cashew butter
2 teaspoons all-fruit jam

(6) 1 cup nonfat plain yogurt (soy yogurt is fine, too)
½ cup berries
¼ cup whole-grain cereal or granola
*You can layer these in a glass or bowl for the parfait effect.*

(7) ¾ cup lowfat cottage cheese
½ cup chopped vegetables (carrots, peppers, tomatoes, etc.)
4 whole-grain crackers

(8) 2 whole-grain toaster waffles
1 tablespoon peanut butter
½ banana

(9) Whole-wheat bagel (small—not the Volkswagen-sized bagels),
schmeer of light cream cheese or tofu cream cheese, with a slice of
tomato or a dollop of jam

## LUNCH

(1) 8 ounces low-sodium vegetarian soup: minestrone, split pea,
vegetable barley, etc.
1½ cups raw mixed greens plus carrots, tomatoes, cukes, radishes,
mushrooms (whatever vegetables you like), 2 ounces tofu or 2 tablespoons chopped nuts or ½ cup beans (chickpeas, kidney beans)

(2) 2 slices whole-wheat bread, 2 tablespoons almond butter,
½ sliced apple
1 cup fat-free milk

(3) ¼ medium sliced avocado in whole-wheat wrap with hummus,
fresh spinach, tomato, sprouts, shredded carrots

(4) Whole-wheat pita stuffed with baked falafel, chopped onions,
tomatoes, and lettuce, 2 teaspoons tahini dressing, hot sauce (optional)

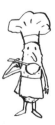

(5) Soy turkey on whole-grain bread with lettuce, tomato, mustard,
side salad

## EATING LUNCH OUT

*Watch portion sizes!*

(1) Chinese
Steamed broccoli, tofu, brown rice (about ½ to ⅔ cup), any sauce on
the side, use sparingly—about 1–2 tablespoons
Moo shu vegetables, sauce on the side, use sparingly
(I know the moo shu pancakes won't be whole grain);
hold the MSG

(2) Mexican
Spinach and mushrooms on a whole-wheat tortilla, with black beans
and corn (no cheese or part-skim cheese; no sour cream)
Small side refried beans (no lard)

(3) Italian
Vegetables (spinach, broccoli, eggplant, mushrooms) on no-cheese
pizza (or low-fat or fat-free cheese if available),
2 regular sized slices

## SNACKS

*Always have a beverage with a snack.*

Baby carrots, celery sticks, hummus (about ¼ cup)
½ apple with 2 teaspoons peanut butter
1 handful of unsalted nuts (about 9–12)
6 ounces nonfat fruit yogurt
1 whole-grain energy bar (no hydrogenated oils, no more than 2 grams
saturated fat per bar)
2 low-fat mini Baby Bell cheese rounds
3 dark chocolate Kisses
¼ cup trail mix (a handful)
Baked tortilla chips (a 1-ounce bag) with salsa
½ ounce Sun Chips (8 chips), 2 tablespoons baba ganoush
or hummus

## DINNER

*On average, vegetables should take up half your plate, healthy protein should take up a quarter, and whole grain should take up the other quarter.*

(1) Pasta primavera—whole-grain pasta with tons of vegetables such as ¼ cup edamame, zucchini, broccoli, onions, carrots, and mushrooms, sautéed with garlic in 1 tablespoon of extra virgin olive oil; add herbs like basil and oregano to taste
Side salad—mixed greens, radishes, carrots, mushrooms, cucumbers, 1 tablespoon dressing

(2) Veggie burger on a whole-grain bun (do not microwave veggie burgers—it makes them taste soggy), dab of no-sodium ketchup or mustard (optional)
Zucchini, lightly sautéed in 2 teaspoons of extra virgin olive oil with garlic and fresh basil, if available, or dried basil

(3) Vegetarian lentil soup (canned or frozen low-sodium is easy to find)
2 slices crusty whole-wheat bread
Chopped vegetable salad (chop mixed greens, radicchio, onions, tomatoes, cucumbers, celery, parsley) with balsamic vinaigrette

(4) Vegetarian chili (you can buy canned, low-sodium), brown-wild rice blend (or just plain brown rice, about ⅔ cup cooked or less), 75 percent light cheddar cheese, shredded, 2 tablespoons
Side salad or lightly steamed broccoli with lemon

## EATING DINNER OUT

### (1) Italian
Eggplant parmesan without the cheese (it is quite good!), broccoli rabe or escarole sautéed in garlic and olive oil—eat half of whatever portion they give you

### (2) Salad bar
Greens, raw or cooked vegetables including carrots, tomatoes, radishes,

celery, mushrooms, a few olives, corn, 3 slices of avocado,
plus ½ cup beans or tofu
1 tablespoon sunflower seeds
2 tablespoons oil and vinegar, vinaigrette, or a squeeze of plain lemon
No potato salad, carrot-raisin salad, egg salad, coleslaw
1 small whole-wheat pita

### (3) Chinese
3 steamed vegetable dumplings (go easy on the dipping sauce), tofu and
vegetable stir fry (light oil), ⅔ cup brown rice

### (4) Indian
Grilled vegetables, raita (this is a yogurt dish and probably will not be
low-fat yogurt, but you can't be perfect all the time), whole-wheat nan,
mulligatawny soup, brown basmati rice (about ⅔ cup) if they have it

### (5) Mexican
Quesadilla (whole wheat if you can get it) stuffed with black beans,
poblano peppers, corn, and grilled onion; no cheese or sour cream; side
of spinach or other mixed vegetables
7–10 tortilla chips (count them—it is easy to eat dozens before you
know it) with salsa and 3 tablespoons of guacamole

### (6) Middle Eastern
Get the platter with hummus, tabouleh, and baba ganoush, whole-
wheat pita; tabouleh is a salad made with couscous, parsley, garlic,
tomatoes, and lemon, and baba ganoush is mashed eggplant with
tahini (sesame paste), lemon, garlic, and spices

## SWEETS 'N' TREATS

Fat-free frozen yogurt, ½ cup
3 dark chocolate Kisses
1 Tofutti chocolate fudge popsicle
1 cup fruit salad
¾ cup unsweetened apple sauce, 1 teaspoon walnuts, pinch of cinnamon
2 Nabisco 100 percent whole-grain Fig Newtons

Low-fat chocolate pudding
½ cup sorbet
1 frozen all-fruit bar

### ALL-DAY BEVERAGES

Water, flavored seltzer, green tea, black tea, herbal teas, unsweetened iced tea, fat-free milk, fat-free hot chocolate (no whip!), coffee or cappuccino with fat-free milk (decaf or regular)

### SALAD DRESSINGS

Use 2 tablespoons:
Vinaigrette
Oil and Vinegar
Fat-free Russian, ranch or blue cheese
Lemon

## Nutrition Prescriptions for Mood, Smarts, Memory, and Focus

### Prescription for a Good Mood

Aside from a colleague losing a presentation you spent days working on or your perfect toddler suddenly hitting the "terrible twos," a bad mood is often generated by low blood sugar, fatigue, hunger, stress, or all of the above. The protein and carbohydrate chapters discuss whole grains and healthy protein options.

- Do not skip meals. Do not go more than three to four hours between meals or snacks. Going too long without food puts your body on alert that it is running out of available fuel. This leads to low blood sugar, which means there is less circulating glucose for your brain. Being Mary Sunshine is not the brain's number one priority, so when blood sugar runs a bit low, the brain will use the available energy for physiological rather than psychological functions. Your smile turns into a grimace and crankiness reigns.

- Go combo. Be sure all meals and snacks are a combination of healthy protein and whole-grain carbohydrates. The protein and carbohydrates work together to provide a sustained release of energy to help prevent your energy and mood from crashing.
- Exercise daily. It may seem impossible to get up and go for a walk when you are feeling blue. But even as little as 10 minutes on a stationary bike can boost your mood, reports a small study of college students in the journal *Health Psychology*. Ten minutes of moderate exercise was enough to improve scores on overall mood and vigor and decrease fatigue. Research shows that regular exercise improves mood and quality of life and reduces depressive symptoms. The Scottish Health Survey, which included almost 20,000 participants, found that 20 minutes of any activity significantly reduced psychological distress. The more the participants exercised, the greater their mental health benefits.

### Good Mood Snack Ideas
- 6 ounces fat-free chocolate milk (or hot chocolate)
- 1 ounce low-fat or nonfat cheese on 1 slice whole-wheat bread
- ½ cup low-fat cottage cheese with ½ cup berries (all are good)
- 1 banana with 2 teaspoons of peanut butter
- 1 tablespoon hummus with ¾ cup baby carrots

## Prescription for Smarts

Start your day with a bright brain. Eat breakfast. Be sure you and your kids eat a healthy breakfast. Go into the cupboard and get rid of the sugar-frosted, chocolate, cookie, honey-dipped cereals (candy in boxes if you ask me) and buy some whole-grain healthier fare. Shredded wheat, oatmeal, Total, Kashi, and other whole-grain cereals are a good morning choice. Add some protein for the morning amino brain bath and you've got a recipe for genius.

- Eating breakfast is associated with significant improvement in student academic performance and psychosocial functioning in children.
- Eating oatmeal boosts kids' cognitive skills better than refined, low-fiber breakfast cereals.

- Eating whole-grain cereals compared with sugary, refined cereals reduces the typical morning decline in attention and memory processes in children.
- One study found that kids eating All-Bran (a high-fiber, whole-grain cereal) did better on attention and memory tests than the kids who ate Cocoa Puffs (low-fiber, refined cereal).
- One study found that men who eat breakfast cereals weigh less and have a lower BMI (body mass index) than men who do not.

## Breakfast Ideas for Brains
- Scrambled egg whites (or Egg Beaters) equal to about 2 eggs; with ¼ cup chopped peppers, ½ cup sliced mushrooms. Cook in a nonstick skillet or a regular skillet with a teaspoon of olive or canola oil. Add pepper to taste. Serve on whole-wheat English muffin dry or with a teaspoon of vegan margarine (I like Earth Balance. It has about half the saturated fat of regular butter).
- 1 cup Kashi cereal topped with ½ cup of blueberries, 1 cup fat-free organic milk, 2 teaspoons chopped walnuts
- Cashew butter on small whole-grain bagel with 2 or 3 sliced strawberries
- 8 ounces fat-free vanilla yogurt, ½ cup raspberries, 2 tablespoons of granola or Grapenuts

## Prescription for Memory

We all get forgetful at times. Stress, fatigue, and poor diet all contribute to memory lapses. Getting your vitamin Bs, omega-3s, and plenty of sleep can help fire up those memory neurons. This prescription was put together using the B foods, omega-3 foods, and sleep tips in Chapters 1, 4, and 5 (I added a few more for fun).

## Memory Food Ideas
- 2 whole-grain waffles topped with nonfat vanilla yogurt and 2 tablespoons ground flaxseeds, a dash of cinnamon
- ½ cup low-fat cottage cheese with ¼ slice of cantaloupe or honeydew melon, 1 teaspoon chopped walnuts

- Breakfast (or anytime) burrito with scrambled eggs—1 yolk, 3 whites; add ¼ cup black or pinto beans; put in a whole-wheat burrito or corn tortilla, top with shredded soy cheese or part-skim mozzarella and salsa to taste.
- 12 ounces low-sodium lentil soup, whole-grain crackers (about 100 calories' worth)
- 4 tablespoons hummus on whole-wheat pita with 2 tablespoons chopped tomatoes, 2 tablespoons chopped celery
- ½ cup vegetarian refried beans, 1 ounce low-fat shredded cheese (75 percent light cheddar would work here); sautéed spinach (1 cup or more cooked), with 1 clove chopped garlic, in 2 teaspoons canola oil
- 3–4 ounces broiled halibut with lemon, herbs like rosemary or thyme, and 1 tablespoon chopped pistachios
- 1–2 cups mixed greens including watercress, 3 ounces canned or grilled salmon, 2 tablespoons vinaigrette, sprinkle of pepper

### Getting a Good Night's Sleep

More than 26 million Americans experience frequent back pain. Being uncomfortable can lead to poor sleep and fatigue. It may be time to get a new mattress. One study found that people who slept on new beds reported a 62.8 percent improvement in lower back pain, 62.4 percent in shoulder pain, 58.4 percent in back stiffness, and 69.5 percent in sleep quality. The Better Sleep Foundation recommends replacing your old mattress every five to seven years for optimal comfort and support.

It is a common belief that a firm mattress is the best for an aching back. But a study in the journal the *Lancet* says differently. In the study 313 people who complained of chronic low back pain had their own bed mattresses replaced with either a firm or a medium-firm mattress. After three months, people who used medium-firm mattresses in the study were twice as likely to report improvements in low back pain than the people who slept on firm mattresses.

### Schmoozing with Your Friends for a Memory Boost

Researchers at the University of Michigan found that 10 minutes of talking to another person can improve memory and test performance in young and older folks alike. The authors contend that e-mail, IMs, and texting don't count. Real social interaction is what seems to make the difference. Call a friend, visit a neighbor, or go out to dinner with your sister to get your daily dose of memory-enhancing schmoozing.

## Prescription for Mental Focus and Clarity

Ever have one of those days where you cannot clear the cobwebs from your brain? You rush out of the house to get the kids to school on time and the next thing you know you are at the gym, with the kids still in the car. This is when a quick mental fix is called for.

- Have a cup of coffee or tea. The caffeine will help amplify your mental focus and clear the fog.
- Eat a high carbohydrate breakfast with some good quality protein. Glucose will give your brain the energy it needs to jump into gear. Protein will supply amino acids for a full quota of neurotransmitters and help manage energy levels.
- Drink water. Being even a little bit dehydrated can suck the energy right out of you. Be sure to hydrate all day long.

**Focus Fuels**
- Coffee
- Tea (has less caffeine than coffee)
- ½ cup dry oatmeal cooked according to package directions, 1 cup fat-free organic milk, ½ apple sliced, dash of cinnamon, 1 teaspoon brown sugar or honey to taste, 2 teaspoons chopped walnuts.
- Whole-wheat English muffin, tofu cream cheese, slice of tomato
- 8 ounces fat-free plain or vanilla yogurt, ½ cup orange juice, ½ cup strawberries, ½ banana, 2 tablespoons wheat germ, 1 teaspoon honey, 1 tablespoon fresh lemon juice, put in blender for a morning smoothie

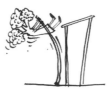

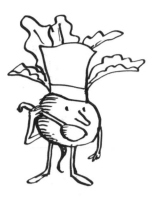

# Recipes You Can Live With

Here is a sampling of fun, healthy recipes for you to try. I was fortunate enough to have these extremely talented chefs share their recipes with me for *Get Smart*. Be sure to check out their cookbooks and Web sites.

## Chefs

**Amie Guyette Hall,** a graduate of the Institute for Integrative Nutrition, is a chef and certified holistic health counselor in Fairfield, Connecticut. She generously donated the bulk of the recipes for this section of the book. Amie teaches children and adults alike how to get back in touch with the land, introduces them to the joys of cooking, and helps them incorporate healthy foods into a healthy lifestyle. She is spearheading programs to get locally grown, healthy foods into local schools as well as writing curriculum for educating kids of all ages about the wonderful benefits of good nutrition. Visit Amie's Web site for more about her and her delicious recipes: www.FromYourInsideOut.com.

**Devin Alexander** is beautiful, talented, and incredibly nice. She is the host of *Healthy Decadence with Devin Alexander* on the Discovery Health channel. She was kind enough to give me recipes from her book *The Most Decadent Diet Ever!* (Broadway Books, 2008). You can find Devin in cyberspace at www.devinalexander.com.

**Missy Chase Lapine,** an innovative and creative chef, is the author of *The Sneaky Chef: Simple Strategies for Hiding Healthy Foods in Kids' Favorite Meals* (Running Press, 2006). She has discovered ways to sneak vegetables into everything from soups to desserts! She is a prolific chef with many more cookbooks on the horizon. Find out what Missy is up to and what her latest books are on her Web site: www.TheSneakyChef.com.

**Rosa J. Donohue, M.S., R.D., C.D.N.,** is a registered dietitian and nutrition consultant with decades of clinical experience working in St. Vincent's Hospital in New York City and consulting in Vermont and New York. Her work in setting up community gardens, nutrition counseling, and cooking classes is ongoing. Rosa's commitment to public service and health education is outstanding.

**Frances Largeman-Roth, M.S., R.D.,** is a registered dietitian and the senior food and nutrition editor at *Health* magazine, where she works on healthy recipes, food trends, weight-loss issues, and the latest nutrition research. She also writes a monthly food and health trend column called "Hot Dish." Frances is the author of *Feed the Belly: The Expectant Mom's Healthy Eating Guide* (Source Books, 2009).

**B. Smith (aka Barbara Smith)** is a former fashion model turned restaurateur, television host, author, entrepreneur, and entertainer and is widely regarded as an expert when it comes to casual but elegant living. B. and I worked together to create these healthy, diabetes-friendly recipes for the Healthy Menu Makeover Program Journey for Control. You can see more at www.JourneyforControl.com.

## Recipes

# *Breakfasts*

### SNEAKY CHEF BONANZA CRUNCH MUFFINS

Missy Chase Lapine, *The Sneaky Chef*

Makes 6 large muffins

| | |
|---:|:---|
| **1** | large egg |
| **¼ cup** | sugar |
| **¼ cup** | almond or canola oil |
| **6 tbs** | Orange Puree (see Make-Ahead Recipe, page 181) |
| **2** | large bananas, mashed with the back of a fork (about ½ cup) |
| **1 tsp** | pure vanilla extract |
| **¾ cup** | flour blend (equal parts white flour, whole wheat flour, and wheat germ) |
| **2 tsp** | baking powder |
| **½ tsp** | cinnamon |
| **½ cup** | oat bran |
| **1½ tsp** | salt |
| **¼ cup** | chopped walnuts, for topping (optional) |

Preheat the oven to 375°. Line a muffin tin with paper liners.

In a large bowl, whisk together the egg and sugar until well combined, then whisk in the oil, Orange Puree, bananas, and vanilla. In another bowl, whisk together the Flour Blend, baking powder, cinnamon, oat bran, and salt. Fold the dry ingredients into the wet, and mix until the flour is just moistened. Don't overmix, or the muffins will be dense.

Fill each muffin cup to the top, spooning about ¼ cup of batter into each. Sprinkle the tops with a few chopped walnuts, if using, and bake for 24–26 minutes, until the tops are golden brown.

## SNEAKY CHEF MAKE-AHEAD RECIPE: ORANGE PUREE
Missy Chase Lapine, *The Sneaky Chef*

Makes about 2 cups of puree

| | |
|---|---|
| **1** | medium sweet potato or yam, peeled and coarsely chopped |
| **3** | medium to large carrots, peeled and sliced into thick chunks |
| **2 to 3 tbs** | water |

In a medium-sized pot, cover the sweet potatoes and carrots with cold water and boil for about 20 minutes, until carrots are very tender. If the carrots aren't thoroughly cooked, they'll leave telltale little nuggets of vegetables in recipes, which will reveal their presence to your man—a gigantic no-no for the Sneaky Chef.

Drain the sweet potatoes and carrots and put them in the food processor with two tablespoons of water. Puree on high until smooth; no pieces of carrots or potatoes should remain. Stop occasionally to push the contents to the bottom. If necessary, use another tablespoon of water to smooth out the puree, but the less water, the better.

This recipe makes about 2 cups of puree; double it if you want to store another 2 cups. It will keep in the refrigerator for up to 3 days, or you can freeze ¼-cup portions in sealed plastic bags or small plastic containers.

## HIGH-FIBER ZUCCHINI BREAKFAST MUFFINS
Rosa J. Donohue, M.S., R.D., C.D.N.

Makes 12 large muffins or 24 mini-muffins

| | |
|---|---|
| **1 cup** | raw quick oatmeal, not instant |
| **1 cup** | whole wheat flour or unbleached flour |
| **3 tbs** | flaxseed meal |
| **2** | eggs |
| **1 tbs** | baking powder |
| **½ tsp** | baking soda |

**½ cup plus 2 level tbs**  brown sugar

**1½ cup**  raw shredded zucchini

**1 cup**  peeled and chopped apples

**½ cup**  soymilk or rice milk

**¼ cup**  *unsweetened* applesauce

grated rind of one large lemon

**½ tsp**  cinnamon

**½ cup**  chopped walnuts or pecans

**¼ cup**  fresh or frozen cranberries, coarsely chopped or cut in half

1. Put shredded zucchini in a colander and let stand 15 minutes while preparing rest of ingredients.

2. Preheat oven to 400°.

3. Grease muffin pans or muffin cups.

4. Mix dry ingredients in a large bowl.

5. Mix all wet ingredients in another bowl.

6. Press zucchini and drain off liquid. Add zucchini, apple and all dry ingredients.

7. Mix well!

8. Spoon batter into cups.

9. Bake for about 20–22 minutes or until muffins are golden brown on top and a toothpick inserted into one comes out clean. If using mini-muffins pan, bake for only 12 minutes, testing with a toothpick also.

10. Cool and serve warm or cold. Cover and refrigerate leftovers.

## STEEL CUT OATS

Amie G. Hall, CHHC, AADP

Serves 1

**1 cup** water
**¼ cup** organic steel cut oats

1. Place water & oats in saucepan.

2. Bring to a boil and reduce heat. Simmer gently for about 20–25 minutes, stirring occasionally to desired thickness.

Tip: Measure water and oats the night before and place in saucepan … letting them soak lessens the cooking time.

Serving suggestions: Make into a complete meal that satisfies tastes and textures that your body craves! Top with maple syrup, agave nectar or honey, then your personalized choice of fruit, fresh or dried … raspberries, blueberries, banana, apple or raisins, cranberries, cherries, you choose. Then go for the protein & healthy fats and oils with the crunch of almonds, walnuts or pecans, pumpkin seeds or sunflower seeds. And of course, remember the cinnamon!

Mix it up: Try adding a little cooked brown rice, millet, or quinoa.

Where to buy: Trader Joe's, Stop & Shop, Shaw's, Hannaford, Whole Foods, and most every health food store.

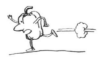

# Sides

## SMOOTHIES
Amie G. Hall, CHHC, AADP

An assortment of healthy smoothies to jump-start your day, to enjoy as
a snack or a creamy, cool dessert.
Assemble ingredients.
Place ingredients into blender.
Blend on high speed until very smooth.

### TROPICAL FREEZE SMOOTHIE
|       |       |
|------:|-------|
| 1 | banana |
| ½ cup | frozen pineapple tidbits |
| ½ cup | frozen mango chunks |
| 1 cup | rice milk or apple cider |
| 6 | ice cubes |

### MY SMOOTHIE
|       |       |
|------:|-------|
| 1 | banana |
| 6 | ice cubes |
| ¼ cup | almond butter |
| Splash | of apple cider |
| 1 tbs | honey or agave nectar |

### COTTON CANDY SMOOTHIE
A bright spring green color and named by my son Weston, age 14.
|       |       |
|------:|-------|
| 2 | bananas |
| ½ cup | frozen pineapple chunks |
| ½ cup | frozen mango chunks (or pineapple) |
| 6–8 | ice cubes |
| 1 | large leaf, leaf only, Swiss chard or bok choy (can add some fresh parsley, too) |
| 2 cups | vanilla rice or almond milk |
| 1–2 tbs | agave nectar (optional) |

## KALE CHIPS

Amie G. Hall, CHHC, AADP

Serves 2–4

**1 bunch** kale
**1 tbs** olive oil
**To taste:** fresh chopped garlic, pepper, curry, cumin, sea salt, gomasio

Preheat oven to 375–400°.

1. Remove kale from the stalk, tearing the greens off in pieces.

2. Place kale in cast iron skillet and drizzle the olive oil over the leaves.

3. Using your hands or tongs, toss the kale about, coating the pieces with the olive oil.

4. Sprinkle with desired seasoning.

5. Place skillet in oven and bake for 5 minutes or until it starts to crisp slightly.

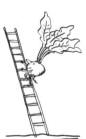

6. Turn kale over and bake the other side until crisp … just 2–3 minutes.

7. Continue to bake until completely crispy.

8. Remove and serve.

9. Eat immediately or cool completely and store in airtight container.

A funky, crunchy snack with hand to mouth satisfaction!

## SNEAKY CHEF NO DOC GUAC
Missy Chase Lapine, *The Sneaky Chef*

Makes about 6 appetizer servings

|  |  |
|--:|:--|
| **2** | ripe avocados |
| | Juice from 1 lime |
| **½ tsp** | salt |
| **¼ to ½ cup** | Green Puree (see Make-Ahead Recipe below) |
| **Optional extra boost:** | ½ cup chopped red onion, chopped tomatoes, handful of chopped cilantro (or fresh basil), and/or chopped jalapeños, to taste |

Halve the avocados lengthwise, remove the pit, and scoop out the flesh. In a small bowl, combine the avocado with the lime juice, salt, Green Puree, and the optional extras, if using. Blend lightly with a fork.

## SNEAKY CHEF MAKE-AHEAD RECIPE: GREEN PUREE
Missy Chase Lapine, *The Sneaky Chef*

Makes about 2 cups of puree

|  |  |
|--:|:--|
| **2 cups** | raw baby spinach leaves |
| **2 cups** | broccoli florets, fresh or frozen |
| **1 cup** | sweet green peas, frozen |
| **2 to 3 tbs** | water |

If using raw spinach, thoroughly wash it, even if the package says "prewashed."

To prepare on the stovetop, pour about 2 inches of water into a pot with a tight-fitting lid. Put a vegetable steamer basket into the pot, add the spinach and broccoli, and steam for about 10 minutes, until very tender. Add the frozen peas to the basket for the last 2 minutes of steaming. Drain.

To prepare in the microwave, place the broccoli and spinach in a microwave-safe bowl, cover with water, and microwave on high for 8 to 10 minutes, until very tender. Add peas for last 2 minutes of cooking. Drain.

Place the vegetables in the bowl of your food processor along with 2 tablespoons of water. Puree on high until as smooth as possible. Stop occasionally to push the contents to the bottom. If necessary, use another tablespoon of water to smooth out the puree.

This recipe makes about 2 cups of puree; double it if you want to store another 2 cups. It will keep in the refrigerator for up to 3 days, or you can freeze ¼-cup portions in sealed plastic bags or small plastic containers.

## STRAWBERRY TOFU FRUIT DIP
Samantha Heller, M.S., R.D., C.D.N.

| | |
|---|---|
| **1 cup** | silken tofu |
| **2 tbs** | maple syrup |
| **½ tsp** | cinnamon |
| **1 tsp** | of 100% vanilla extract |
| **1 cup** | fresh or frozen strawberries (you can use any berries) |

Combine all ingredients in blender and blend until smooth. Add more tofu for a thicker consistency. Use as a dip for sliced fruit.

## WHITE BEAN DIP
Samantha Heller, M.S., R.D., C.D.N.

So easy and delicious

| | |
|---|---|
| **1 15-oz can** | organic cannellini beans |
| **2 tbs** | olive oil |
| **2** | cloves garlic, minced |
| **2–3 tbs** | fresh lemon juice (start with 2 and add a third to taste) |
| **¼ tsp** | kosher salt |
| **2 tsp** | minced fresh rosemary |
| | white pepper to taste |
| | whole-wheat pitas, small |

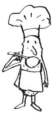

1. Rinse and drain the beans and put into the food processor.

2. Add the olive oil, garlic, lemon juice, salt, and minced rosemary. Puree until the dip has reached the consistency you want. You can add a little water to make it thinner.

3. Pour into serving dish and garnish with a sprig of fresh rosemary and lemon wedge.

4. Drizzle a few drops of olive oil on top.

5. Serve with toasted whole-wheat pita wedges, baby carrots, celery sticks, zucchini. Buy whole-wheat pitas, slice into wedges. Put under broiler until lightly toasted (keep an eye out so they do not burn).

# Salads

## ARAME SLAW
Amie G. Hall, CHHC, AADP

| | |
|---:|---|
| **½-¾ cup** | dried arame sea vegetable, softened (Place arame in small bowl and add water to cover, then let soak to soften. Set aside at least 15 minutes.) |
| **3** | carrots, grated by hand or in food processor |
| **¼** | head of cabbage, coarsely chopped (white or purple) |
| **3-4** | scallions, thin sliced on diagonal |
| **¼ cup or more** | sesame seeds, gently toasted in dry skillet |
| **½ cup** | sliced almonds, gently toasted in dry skillet (optional) |
| **1 tbs** | brown rice vinegar |
| **2-3 tbs** | toasted sesame oil |
| **2 tsp** | agave nectar |
| | Sea salt, to taste |

Combine softened arame, carrot, cabbage, scallion, sesame seeds and almonds in bowl.

In separate small bowl lightly whisk together the vinegar, oil, agave and sea salt with fork or small whisk.

Pour dressing over mixture and toss lightly.

**Kitchen Freedom Tip:** Hiziki sea vegetable also works well. Feel free to add in more scallion or adjust any of the above quantities. Sesame seeds and almonds are optional, but really bring balance and satisfaction to this crisp, refreshing salad!

## PINTO BEAN SPREAD (REFRIED BEANS)
Amie G. Hall, CHHC, AADP

| | |
|---|---|
| **2 15-oz cans** | pinto beans, or light or red kidney beans, undrained |
| **3–4** | cloves garlic, finely chopped |
| **½** | red onion, chopped |
| **½** | red pepper, chopped |
| **2 tbs** | olive oil |
| **1 tbs** | cumin |
| **1 pinch** | cayenne or chipotle pepper, to taste |
| | sea salt & fresh ground pepper |

1. In large skillet, sauté garlic, onion and red pepper in olive oil until soft.

2. Add the pinto beans, or light or red kidney beans, 1 tbs cumin, 1 pinch cayenne or chipotle pepper, to taste, sea salt & fresh ground pepper.

3. Add 1 can water and cook on low for quite a while. Add more water as needed, until beans are very tender and there is no more liquid.

4. To finish, mash mixture with a fork for a chunky bean paste or puree in food processor until smooth.

5. Sprinkle with fresh chopped cilantro.

6. Serve with tortilla chips or in a wrap. Substitute in place of canned refried beans.

## QUINOA SALAD WITH PORTOBELLO & PARMESAN
Amie G. Hall, CHHC, AADP

Serves about 8

| | |
|---|---|
| **2 cups** | quinoa |
| **4 cups** | water |
| **1** | large Portobello mushroom or 6–8 baby Portobello mushrooms |
| **1** | small yellow onion |
| **½ cup** | sundried tomato, finely chopped or snipped with scissors |
| **½ cup** | fresh basil leaves, chopped (can substitute cilantro or dill) |
| **2–3** | cloves garlic, peeled, minced |
| **¼ cup** | freshly grated parmesan cheese |
| **⅓ cup** | olive oil, plus 2–3 tbs for sautéing. |
| **1 tbs** | balsamic vinegar |
| **¼ tsp** | sea salt & pepper |

1. Put quinoa & water in medium saucepan and place on burner on medium to high heat. Bring to boil and reduce heat. Cook gently, about 10–12 minutes until done and set aside in large bowl.

2. Sauté 1 large Portobello mushroom (gills removed), or 6–8 baby Portobello mushrooms, sliced and finely chopped, in olive oil on medium to high heat. Add to bowl.

3. Chop 1 small yellow onion and sauté in olive oil until translucent & nicely caramelized. To finish, deglaze pan by adding a splash of balsamic vinegar to the onions and bring to a boil. Let bubble a few minutes until liquid is almost gone. Add to bowl.

4. Add the sundried tomato, fresh basil leaves, garlic, parmesan cheese to bowl.

5. Stir in ⅓ cup olive oil and add sea salt & pepper to taste.

6. Serve as a warm pilaf or as a cold salad.

## SOUTHWEST QUINOA SALAD
Amie G. Hall, CHHC, AADP

Serves 8–10

| | |
|---|---|
| **1 15-oz can** | black beans, drained and rinsed |
| **2 cups** | cooked quinoa, prepared according to directions on box (any other favorite cooked grain may be substituted such as brown rice, millet, wheat berries) |
| **2 cups** | diced mango, or pineapple or papaya or a combo of (use fresh or frozen, thawed) |
| **1 cup** | diced red pepper |
| **6** | green onions, thinly sliced and chopped |
| **¼ cup** | red onion, chopped |
| **¼ cup** | cilantro leaves, chopped (could substitute mint leaves) |
| **1** | lime, juiced |
| **2 tbs** | olive oil |
| **1** | jalapeno, seeded and minced |
| | Sea salt to taste |

1. Combine ingredients in bowl.

2. Toss and serve.

## SPELT SALAD WITH CARROT, PARSNIP, DRIED CHERRY & PECANS

Amie G. Hall, CHHC, AADP

Serves 6–8

| | |
|---:|---|
| **1 cup** | spelt grain (or other whole grain such as brown rice or kamut) |
| **2 cups** | water |
| **1** | carrot |
| **1** | parsnip |
| **1 cup** | pecan halves |
| **½–¾ cup** | dried cherry or cranberry |
| **¼ cup** | red onion, minced |
| **¼ cup** | chopped fresh mint |
| **¼ cup** | toasted sesame seed oil, plus 1 tbs for cooking Sea salt & pepper to taste |

1. Cook the spelt grain in water until liquid is absorbed and set aside in mixing bowl.

2. Wash well and do not peel carrot and parsnip. Cut ends off each and cut in half lengthwise, then in quarters. Sauté the carrot & parsnip in 1 tbs toasted sesame seed oil until lightly golden and slightly tender. Add to bowl.

3. Slice celery lengthwise in half or thirds and chop in small chunks and add to bowl.

4. Add pecans, dried cherry or cranberry, red onion, & mint to bowl. Stir all ingredients with spoon.

5. Add sesame oil, sea salt & pepper, to taste.

6. Serve room temperature, cold or heated.

## BLACK-EYED PEA SALAD
B. Smith

| | |
|---:|:---|
| **3 tbs** | extra virgin olive oil |
| **2 tbs** | balsamic vinegar |
| **1 ¼ tsp** | ground cumin |
| **1 ¼ tsp** | minced garlic |
| **¾ tsp** | salt |
| **½ tsp** | cayenne pepper |
| **¼ cup** | finely chopped red onion |
| **½ cup** | chopped red bell pepper |
| **2 tbs** | chopped black olives |
| **3 tbs** | chopped fresh basil leaves |
| **2 tbs** | chopped pimentos |
| **2 cups** | cooked brown rice or whole wheat pasta |
| **2 cups** | cooked fresh or frozen black-eyed peas |
| **8 cups** | salad greens |

In a large bowl, whisk together the olive oil, vinegar, cumin, garlic, salt and cayenne pepper. Add the onion, bell pepper, olives, basil, pimentos, rice and peas. Toss the salad enough to moisten. Cover and refrigerate up to 24 hours. Serve on a bed of salad greens.

# *Lunch*

## BLACK BEAN SOUP

Amie G. Hall, CHHC, AADP

Serves 6–8

| | |
|---:|---|
| **2 cups** | dried black beans, soaked |
| **1** | onion, chopped |
| **4** | cloves garlic, crushed & minced |
| **½ cup** | red pepper, chopped |
| **1** | large carrot, chopped |
| **1** | stalk celery, chopped |
| **2 quarts** | vegetable stock (two 1-quart boxes or homemade) |
| **2" piece** | kombu seaweed (Kombu helps to soften the beans during cooking and can be found in the Asian section of most food stores.) |
| **2 tbs** | olive oil |
| **2 tsp** | sea salt |
| **1** | orange |
| | black pepper, & cayenne or chipotle pepper to taste |

1. Soak black beans covered in water overnight or for at least 4 hours.

Soaking your beans releases phytic acid and helps to ease digestive concerns. Discard water* and rinse beans.

2. Sauté in soup pot: onion, garlic, red pepper.

3. Add carrot & celery and continue cooking, stirring until tender, about 10 minutes.

4. Add beans to soup pot with vegetable stock, the kombu & sea salt.

Bring to a boil and let simmer 1–2 hours on low heat.

5. Add juice of one whole orange, optional.

6. Add fresh black pepper and cayenne or chipotle pepper to add heat, to taste. Continue cooking 10 minutes on low.

7. Check soup and ask yourself if this soup suits you. Is it too thick, add some water or more stock. Do you want it thicker, heartier? Silkier and smoother? Puree with a hand blender or food processor. Want it hotter? Add more pepper.

8. Top with freshly chopped red onion, cilantro or chives. Enjoy!

About 2 hours cooking time, not including bean soaking time.
Need a short cut? Use two 25 ounce cans of black beans.

*Use bean water to water plants or garden!

## TANGY GAZPACHO
B. Smith

| | |
|---|---|
| 3 ½ | cups seeded peeled ripe tomatoes (about 2 pounds)· |
| 1 cup | chopped, seeded, peeled cucumber (½ medium) |
| 1 cup | chopped red bell pepper |
| 1 cup | chopped green bell pepper |
| ½ cup | chopped red onion |
| ½ cup | chopped carrots |
| ¼ cup | chopped celery |
| ¼ cup | fresh cilantro leaves |
| 1 tsp | chopped garlic |
| 2 tbs | olive oil |
| 2 tbs | cider vinegar |
| 1 tbs | fresh lime juice |

| | |
|---|---|
| **½ tsp** | paprika |
| **1 tsp** | salt |
| **¼ tsp** | ground black pepper |
| **¼ tsp** | ground cumin |
| **⅛ tsp** | cayenne pepper |
| **1 ½ cups** | tomato juice (low sodium) |
| | Fresh cilantro leaves for garnish |

Place the tomatoes, cucumber, bell peppers, onion, carrots, celery, cilantro leaves and garlic in a food processor. Add the oil, vinegar and lime juice. Puree until smooth.

## CALIFORNIA OPEN-FACE SANDWICH
Samantha Heller, M.S., R.D., C.D.N.

| | |
|---|---|
| **1 slice** | 100% whole-grain bread |
| **¼** | ripe avocado sliced |
| **2** | thin slices fresh tomato |
| **1 tbs** | chopped sweet onion |
| **1 oz** | shredded soy cheddar cheese or 75% light cheddar cheese |
| | Sprinkling of sesame seeds |
| **2 tsp** | balsamic vinaigrette |

Layer ingredients on the bread starting with the avocado, tomato, onion, top with cheese and sesame seeds. Drizzle dressing over sandwich. Place under broiler for 3–5 minutes, until cheese is melted.

## CLASSIC PB & B
Samantha Heller, M.S., R.D., C.D.N.

| | |
|---|---|
| **2 slices** | 100% whole-grain bread |
| **2 tbs** | of smooth or crunchy peanut butter (no salt or sugar added) |
| **½** | banana sliced |
| **1 tsp** | honey |
| **Dash** | of cinnamon |

Spread one slice of the bread with the peanut butter. Top with bananas and a drizzle (about a teaspoon) of honey. Add a dash of cinnamon. Put second slice of bread on top. Cut in half. This sandwich travels well.

You can substitute apple or pear slices for the banana.

## ROASTED CAULIFLOWER AND BUTTERNUT SQUASH SOUP
Frances Largeman-Roth, M.S., R.D.

| | |
|---:|---|
| **1 tbs** | olive oil, divided |
| **1** | medium head golden cauliflower, cut into florets |
| **1** | medium butternut squash, peeled, seeded, and cubed |
| **2** | shallots, quartered |
| **2** | large garlic cloves, minced |
| **½ tsp** | salt |
| **½ tsp** | freshly ground black pepper |
| **32 oz** | low-sodium vegetable broth |
| **2 tsp** | fresh thyme |
| **2 cups** | 1% or fat-free organic milk or plain unsweetened soy milk |
| | Additional salt and pepper, to taste |
| **1 tbs** | grated Parmesan cheese |

1. Preheat oven to 350°.

2. Drizzle half of the oil in a roasting pan. Add the cauliflower, squash, shallots, and garlic. Drizzle with the remaining olive oil. Sprinkle on the salt and pepper, and roast for 35 minutes.

3. Transfer the vegetables to a large stock pot, and add the broth and the thyme. Bring to a simmer and cook for 30 minutes until both the cauliflower and squash are very tender.

4. Working in batches, puree ⅔ of the soup mixture in a blender. Remove the middle piece of plastic in the blender lid and cover opening

with a clean cloth—this will allow the steam to escape. Transfer the puree to a bowl and return to the pot when you're finished.

5. Stir in the milk until the consistency is creamy. Add additional salt and pepper to taste, and stir in the Parmesan. Serve while hot.

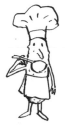

# *Entrees*

### CHICKEN PASTA WITH VODKA CREAM SAUCE
Devin Alexander, *The Most Decadent Diet Ever!*

I created this recipe at the request of one of my celebrity clients. She was trying to lose weight for a movie and swore she kept having nightmares about having overeaten pasta with vodka sauce. She thought I wouldn't be able to redesign it because it's a cream-based sauce. But I managed to quell her craving—and her nightmares. I also suggested she add some chicken to the dish. Though I don't believe any foods are "bad," it's always great to add bulk to your meals with lean protein, especially when you're trying to build muscle. Who knew vodka and looking buff could go hand in hand?

| | |
|---|---|
| **1½ cups** | Vodka Cream Sauce (recipe follows) |
| **8 oz** | dried enriched multigrain rotini or penne pasta |
| **12 oz** | boneless, skinless chicken breast, visible fat removed, cut into ¾-inch-wide strips |
| **1½ tsp** | extra virgin olive oil |
| | Salt and pepper |
| **2 tsp** | grated reduced-fat Parmesan |
| **4 tbs** | slivered fresh basil leaves, or to taste |

Prepare the Vodka Cream Sauce. Cook the pasta according to package directions.

Toss the chicken and olive oil in a small bowl, and season with salt and pepper to taste.

Place a medium nonstick skillet over medium-high heat. When the skillet is hot, put in the chicken and cook until browned on the outside and no longer pink inside, about 3 minutes per side.

Drain the pasta and divide it among 4 medium shallow bowls. Spoon a quarter of the sauce into the center of each. Top each bowl with a quarter of the chicken. Then sprinkle a quarter of the Parmesan and basil leaves evenly over the top of each bowl. Serve immediately.

Makes 4 servings

Each 4-Decadent-Disk serving (¼ recipe) has: 401 calories, 33 g protein, 50 g carbohydrates, 6 g fat, <1 g saturated fat, 55 mg cholesterol, 6 g fiber, 349 mg sodium.

## VODKA CREAM SAUCE

Vodka cream sauce does have vodka in it, but not a lot. It's actually a creamy tomato sauce with the mildest hint of vodka. When you make this, I implore you to chop the garlic yourself—the stuff in the jar just won't give you the same flavor. If you're short on time, just buy the peeled cloves that are now found in the produce section of most major grocery stores. They can be chopped in seconds.

| | |
|---:|:---|
| **1 tsp** | extra virgin olive oil |
| **1 cup** | minced sweet onions |
| **1 tbs** | minced or crushed fresh garlic |
| **1 28-oz can** | crushed tomatoes |
| **⅓ cup** | vodka |
| **1 cup** | fat-free half-and-half |
| **2 tsp** | fresh lemon juice |
| **¼ cup plus 2 tbs** | reduced-fat Parmesan |
| **½ tsp** | dried basil |
| **½ tsp** | dried oregano |
| **1 tsp** | sugar |
| **¼ tsp** | salt |

Place a medium nonstick saucepan over medium heat. Put in the olive oil, onions, and garlic and cook, stirring occasionally, until the onions and garlic are sweating and tender but not at all browned, 8 to 10 minutes.

Reduce the heat to low. Add the tomatoes and vodka. Slowly stir in the half-and-half. Then stir in the lemon juice, Parmesan, basil, oregano, sugar, and salt until smooth and well combined. Cook over the lowest heat setting, covered, for at least 3 hours, stirring occasionally. Serve immediately, or refrigerate in an airtight container for up to 5 days.

Makes approximately 4 cups; 8 servings

Each ½-cup serving has: 111 calories, 4 g protein, 15 g carbohydrates, 2 g fat, trace saturated fat, 7 mg cholesterol, 2 g fiber, 332 mg sodium.

### GRILLED CHICKEN WITH BRUSCHETTA TOPPING
Devin Alexander, *The Most Decadent Diet Ever!*

You've probably been to plenty of parties where bruschetta has been served. It's that crisped bread with the wonderfully garlicky fresh tomatoes on top. Well, here's a twist on that. It makes for a super-lean meal full of great muscle-building protein and cancer-preventing tomatoes, with tons of flavor and only heart-healthy fats. It's particularly great for a summer day when fresh tomatoes are in season and thus tend to be less expensive and even more delicious.

| | |
|---:|:---|
| **1 recipe** | Bruschetta Topping (recipe follows) |
| **four 4½-oz** | boneless, skinless chicken breasts, visible fat removed |
| **1 tsp** | extra virgin olive oil |
| **1½ tsp** | minced fresh garlic |
| | Salt and pepper |

Prepare the Bruschetta Topping.

Preheat a grill to high.

Place the chicken breasts between two sheets of plastic wrap or wax paper on a flat work surface. Use the flat side of a meat mallet to pound them to an even ½-inch thickness.

Transfer the chicken to a medium bowl. Add the olive oil and garlic. Mix with your hands until well combined. Season generously with salt and pepper to taste.

Place the chicken breasts side by side on the grill. Turn the heat to medium, if possible, and grill for 3 to 5 minutes per side, until no longer pink inside. Transfer to a platter or individual plates and spoon a quarter of the Bruschetta Topping (about ¼ cup) over each. Serve immediately.

## BRUSCHETTA TOPPING

Makes 1 to 1¼ cups; 4 servings

| | |
|---:|:---|
| 1⅓ cups | seeded and finely chopped Roma tomatoes |
| 1 tbs | finely slivered fresh basil leaves |
| 1 tbs | extra virgin olive oil |
| 1½ tsp | balsamic vinegar |
| 1 tsp | minced or crushed fresh garlic |
| ½ tsp | sugar |
| ¼ tsp | salt |
| Pinch | of black pepper, or to taste |

Mix the tomatoes, basil, olive oil, vinegar, garlic, sugar, salt, and pepper in a medium resealable container. Seal the container and refrigerate for at least 2 hours to let the flavors meld. Serve cold or at room temperature.

Each 2-tablespoon serving has: 23 calories, <1 g protein, 2 g carbohydrates, 2 g fat, <1 g saturated fat, 0 mg cholesterol, <1 g fiber, 75 mg sodium.

Each 2-Decadent-Disk serving (1 chicken breast plus ¼ recipe Bruschetta Topping) has: 199 calories, 30 g protein, 4 g carbohydrates, 6 g fat, 1 g saturated fat, 74 mg cholesterol, <1 g fiber, 232 mg sodium.

## PESTO PARMESAN–CRUSTED SALMON

Devin Alexander, *The Most Decadent Diet Ever!*

Have you ever made pesto? It's astounding how much olive oil will soak into the herbs. Couple that with the fact that most pesto has pine nuts in it, and you have a sauce that is high in fat.

I used to eat pesto all of the time until I realized that. After years of missing it, I started creating what I called "almost-pesto" that I could use as part of a dish to eliminate the excess oil. This "almost-pesto" dish quickly became one of my favorites.

It's very important that the basil leaves are dry before you add them to the food processor. This way you'll ensure the perfect crispy topping.

|  |  |
|---:|:---|
| | Olive oil spray |
| **Four 3½-oz** | skinless salmon fillets, bones removed |
| | Salt and pepper |
| **1** | slice whole-wheat bread |
| **14** | medium fresh basil leaves |
| **1** | medium garlic clove |
| **1 tbs** | grated reduced-fat Parmesan |

Preheat the oven to 400°F.

Lightly mist a small nonstick baking sheet with spray.

Season both sides of the salmon fillets with salt and pepper to taste.

Tear the bread into large pieces and put it in the bowl of a food processor fitted with a chopping blade. Add the basil, garlic, and Parmesan. Process until minced, about 1 minute. Transfer to a sheet of wax paper. Place one fillet on the crumbs, so the side that had the skin is face up. Press it into the crumbs to coat the bottom only. Flip it and place it on the prepared baking sheet, crumb side up. Repeat with the remaining 3 fillets, coating them and then placing them side by side, not touching, on the sheet. If crumbs remain, spoon them among the fillets, and then press them on. Bake, uncovered, for 10 to 12 minutes, or until the fillets are pale pink throughout. Serve immediately.

Can be made in 30 minutes or less / No more than 20 minutes hands-on prep time

Makes 4 servings

Each 2-Decadent-Disk serving (1 fillet) has: 209 calories, 21 g protein, 5 g carbohydrates, 11 g fat, 2 g saturated fat, 60 mg cholesterol, <1 g fiber, 127 mg sodium.

## PAN-SEARED CATFISH
B. Smith

| | |
|---:|:---|
| **4 (8-ounce)** | catfish fillets |
| **1** | egg |
| **½ tsp** | hot pepper sauce |
| **½ cup** | corn meal |
| **2 tsp** | paprika |
| **1 tsp** | ground black pepper |
| **½ tsp** | garlic powder |
| **½ tsp** | onion powder |
| **½ tsp** | low-sodium poultry seasoning |
| **1 tbs** | olive or canola oil |
| | Lemon wedges |

Rinse the fillets and pat them dry with paper towels. In a shallow dish, beat egg and hot pepper sauce until well mixed.

In another shallow dish, stir together corn meal, paprika, black pepper, garlic powder, onion powder and low-sodium poultry seasoning. Dip both sides of fish pieces into egg mixture, then coat with corn meal mixture.

In 12-inch non-stick skillet, heat oil over medium heat until hot. Pan sear fish for 3–4 minutes per side, turning once, until fish flakes easily with fork and is brown on both sides. Drain on paper towels.

To keep underside of fish crisp, immediately place fillets on cooling rack until serving time. Serve with wedges of fresh lemon.

## GLORIOUS GREENS
Amie G. Hall, CHHC, AADP

Select ANY green leafy vegetable when at the market: kale, collards, spinach, Swiss chard, mustard greens, broccoli rabe, dandelion greens, beet greens, arugula, watercress, etc. I like to have 2 or 3 on hand.
Per person:

> Choose 1–2 large leaves or 1 handful of smaller leaf greens

In medium sauté pan, put ¼–½ inch water & place on burner on high heat. When it comes to a boil, add in chopped greens. Sprinkle with a little sea salt. Toss quickly with tongs. Pour off extra water. (Add water to soup if you like.) Drizzle a little olive oil on greens and serve!

*For added nutrients:* Add a splash of tamari or Bragg's Liquid Aminos. Add cashews and dried cherries or white raisins, or pine nuts and tomato. Add chopped garlic and fresh herbs.

For more variety and fun, choose a combination of greens from your fridge.

For example:

1 leaf collard greens, 4 stems broccolini, small handful baby spinach or

1–2 leaves kale, 3 asparagus spears, 1 leaf collard greens

*Choose from what you have on hand. Choose what you want to have.*
*Discover what your favorites are!*
*Small amounts of greens can be added into your scrambled eggs, tomato sauce and soups,*
*and even the kids' mac & cheese!*
*Try to sneak them in wherever you can for the added benefits!!*

## VEGETABLE PAELLA
Rosa J. Donohue, M.S., R.D., C.D.N., Nutrition Consultant

(If you prefer, you can use other types of vegetables or use only what you have available, even frozen vegetables.)

| | |
|---|---|
| **¼ cup** | fresh green beans |
| **¼ cup** | fresh broccoli flowerets |
| **¼ cup** | cauliflower flowerets |
| **½ cup** | firm tofu, drained and cut into small cubes |
| **½** | small red or green bell pepper, diced |
| **2 tbs** | olive or canola oil |
| **½** | small red onion, chopped |
| **1 cup** | cooked brown rice |
| **⅛ tsp** | salt, pepper to taste |
| **1 tsp** | oregano |
| **1 cup** | tomato sauce |
| **½ cup** | cooked chickpeas |
| **2** | cloves garlic, minced |
| **1 tsp** | paprika (optional) |
| **1 tbs** | chopped cilantro or parsley (optional) |
| **2 tbs** | raisins (optional) |
| **5** | pitted, chopped olives (optional) |
| **pinch** | of cayenne pepper |

1. Cook green beans, broccoli and cauliflower (or frozen vegetables) in enough boiling water to cover them, about 3–4 minutes or until crisp-tender; drain.

2. Heat oil in 10-inch skillet over medium-high heat. Put in the garlic, paprika, onions, and red or green pepper and stir for one minute.

3. Add tofu cubes, salt and pepper and cook stirring for 2 minutes.

4. Add other vegetables and stir to mix everything well.

5. Add tomato sauce and cook 2–3 minutes.

6. Stir in remaining ingredients. Cook about 4 minutes, stirring frequently but gently, until hot.

7. Sprinkle chopped cilantro or parsley at the end just before serving.

# Desserts

## APPLE BROWNIE
Rosa J. Donohue, M.S., R.D., C.D.N., Nutrition Consultant

| | |
|---|---|
| ½ cup | unsweetened cocoa powder |
| ⅓ cup | unbleached flour |
| ½ cup | whole wheat flour |
| ½ cup | unsweetened applesauce |
| ¼ tsp | salt |
| 1 tsp | vanilla extract |
| 3 tbs | flaxseed meal (ground flaxseeds) |
| 1 cup | sugar |
| 2 | large egg whites |
| ½ cup | chopped walnuts |
| ¼ cup | raisins (optional) |
| 1 tsp | baking powder |
| 2 tbs | canola oil |

Preheat oven to 350°. Spray or oil 8 x 8 inch pan.

Mix together cocoa powder, flour, baking powder and salt.

In separate bowl, cream sugar and oil, whisk in egg whites, applesauce and vanilla and flaxseed meal.

Spoon flour mixture slowly into the egg mixture and stir only until combined.

Pour into baking pan. Bake for 35–40 minutes until firm to the touch. Do not overcook. These brownies are moist if not left in oven too long. Cool before cutting into squares. You can sprinkle with powder sugar when cool.

You can also use mini-muffins baking pans (about 1 to 1½ inch size muffins) and put a piece of walnut on top of each before baking. It will only take about 10 minutes to bake the tiny muffins, or 15–20 minutes if you use regular size muffin pans.

If you want brownies to be more like fudge, use 2 tablespoons less of the whole wheat flour. Recipe can be doubled easily.

**BROWNIES**
Amie G. Hall, CHHC, AADP

Prep Time: 10 minutes
Cooking Time: 35–45 minutes
Yields: 32 small brownies

| | |
|---|---|
| **1½ cups** | organic chocolate chips (You can also use grain-sweetened, vegan or carob semisweet chocolate chips.) |
| **2 cups** | black beans*, one 25-oz can, drained and rinsed |
| **4** | eggs |
| **2/3 cup** | agave nectar |
| **½ tsp** | baking powder |

*Chickpeas or pinto beans may be substituted for the black beans.

1. In a small bowl melt chips in microwave for 2 minutes. Or place chips in a heat-resistant bowl on top of a pot of boiling water until melted.

2. In blender or food processor with fitted metal blade, process beans until very smooth.

3. Add eggs and process until well blended.

4. Add sweetener, baking powder, and melted chips. Process until smooth.

5. Pour batter into one 9 X 13 pan or two 8" or 9" square pans sprayed with organic olive oil or greased with butter.

6. Bake at 350° for 35–45 minutes.

Allow to cool, cut and serve.

Or cool slightly, and for a more decadent chocolate brownie make the Chocolate Brownie Glaze (below) and spread evenly on brownies:

## CHOCOLATE BROWNIE GLAZE

| | |
|---|---|
| **1 cup** | organic chocolate chips (or other) |
| **¼ cup** | soy, rice or almond milk, original or vanilla flavored |
| **2 tsp** | maple syrup or agave nectar |

1. Melt chips in microwave or in double boiler on stove.

2. Stir in milk and sweetener until smooth & glossy.

3. Spread on warm or cooled brownies. Top with chopped nuts, dried cranberries, raisins, or coconut optional.

**Note:** Gluten-Free

## CHOCOLATE TOFU MOUSSE WITH FRESH RASPBERRIES
Amie G. Hall, CHHC, AADP

Serves 6–8

**1¼ lbs**  silken tofu
**¾ cup**  semisweet organic, vegan or grain-sweetened
chocolate chips, melted

1. In a small bowl melt chips in microwave for 2 minutes. Or place chips in a heat-resistant bowl on top of a pot of boiling water until melted.

2. In a blender: Puree the tofu to a smooth paste.

3. Add the melted chocolate and blend thoroughly.

4. Pour the mousse into six or more dessert glasses or bowls and chill for at least 1–2 hours. Can be made the morning of or day before and let chill several hours or overnight.

5. Top with fresh raspberries & enjoy!

Note: I have also used soft tofu in place of the silken, you just need to blend it longer in the beginning. Give it a try, too.

Also, we find the mousse made with semisweet organic chips (made with organic cane sugar) is definitely sweeter than when made with the grain-sweetened chips. If using grain-sweetened, perhaps add in a little agave nectar.

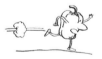

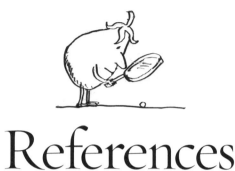

# References

## Introduction

Ferri CP, Prince M, Brayne C, et al. Global prevalence of dementia: a Delphi consensus study. Lancet 2005;366:2112–7.

Fratiglioni L, Paillard-Borg S, Winblad B. An active and socially integrated lifestyle in late life might protect against dementia. Lancet Neurology 2004;3:343–53.

Kaplan RJ, Greenwood CE, Winocur G, Wolever TMS. Cognitive performance is associated with glucose regulation in healthy elderly persons and can be enhanced with glucose and dietary carbohydrates. Am J Clin Nutr 2000;72:825–36.

King DE, Mainous IAG, Geesey ME. Turning back the clock: adopting a healthy lifestyle in middle age. Am J Med 2007;120:598–603.

Liu J, Raine A, Venables PH, Mednick SA. Malnutrition at age 3 years and externalizing behavior problems at ages 8, 11, and 17 years. Am J Psychiat 2004;161:2005–13.

Pfizer Australia. Pfizer Australia Health Report. Looking at dementia: Pfizer Australia Pty Ltd. www.healthreport.com.au/; 2008. Report no. 40.

Small GW, Silverman DHS, Siddarth P, et al. Effects of a 14-day healthy longevity lifestyle program on cognition and brain function. Am J Geriat Psychiat 2006;14:538–45.

# Chapter 1

Alavanja MC, Field RW, Sinha R, et al. Lung cancer risk and red meat consumption among Iowa women. Lung Cancer 2001;34:37–46.

Alzheimer's Disease Fact Sheet. 2006. http://www.nia.nih.gov/Alzheimers/Publications/adfact.htm.

American Cancer Society Guidelines on Diet and Cancer Prevention. American Cancer Society, 1997. http://www.cancer.org/docroot/MED/content/MED_2_1X_American_Cancer_Society_guidelines_on_diet_and_cancer_prevention.asp.

American Heart Association, American Stroke Association. Heart Disease and Stroke Statistics—2008 Update. Our Guide to Current Statistics and the Supplement to Our Heart and Stroke Facts. Dallas: American Heart Association, American Stroke Association; 2008.

Barberger-Gateau P, Letenneur L, Deschamps V, Peres K, Dartigues J-F, Renaud S. Fish, meat, and risk of dementia: cohort study. Brit Med J 2002;325:932–3.

Booyens J, Louwrens CC, Katzeff IE. The role of unnatural dietary trans and cis unsaturated fatty acids in the epidemiology of coronary artery disease. Med Hypotheses 1988;25:175–82.

Bouwstra H, Dijck-Brouwer J, Decsi T, et al. Neurologic condition of healthy term infants at 18 months: positive association with venous umbilical DHA status and negative association with umbilical trans-fatty acids. Pediatr Res 2006;60:334–9.

Chao AP, Thun MJMDMS, Connell CJMPH, et al. Meat consumption and risk of colorectal cancer. JAMA 2005;293:172–82.

Chavarro JE, Rich-Edwards JW, Rosner BA, Willett WC. Dietary fatty acid intakes and the risk of ovulatory infertility. Am J Clin Nutr 2007;85:231–7.

Connor WE. Importance of n-3 fatty acids in health and disease. Am J Clin Nutr 2000;71:171S–5S.

Daviglus ML, Stamler J, Orencia AJ, et al. Fish consumption and the 30-year risk of fatal myocardial infarction. [See comment.] New Engl J Med 1997;336:1046–53.

Davis BC, Kris-Etherton PM. Achieving optimal essential fatty acid status in vegetarians: current knowledge and practical implications. Am J Clin Nutr 2003;78:640S–6S.

de Lau LMLM, Bornebroek MMDP, Witteman JCMP, Hofman AMDP, Koudstaal PJMDP, Breteler MMBMDP. Dietary fatty acids and the risk of Parkinson disease: the Rotterdam Study. Neurology 2005;64:2040–5.

De Vriese SR, Christophe AB, Maes M. In humans, the seasonal variation in polyunsaturated fatty acids is related to the seasonal variation in violent suicide and serotonergic markers of violent suicide. Prostag Leukotr Ess 2004;71:13–8.

The Diabetes Food Pyramid: Fat. www.diabetes.org/nutrition-and-recipes/nutrition/fat.jsp.

Dijck-Brouwer DAJ, Hadders-Algra M, Bouwstra H, et al. Lower fetal status of docosahexaenoic acid, arachidonic acid and essential fatty acids is associated with less favorable neonatal neurological condition. Prostag Leukotr Ess 2005;72:21–8.

Droge W, Schipper HM. Oxidative stress and aberrant signaling in aging and cognitive decline. Aging Cell 2007;6:361–70.

Elias SL, Innis SM. Infant plasma trans, n-6, and n-3 fatty acids and conjugated linoleic acids are related to maternal plasma fatty acids, length of gestation, and birth weight and length. Am J Clin Nutr 2001;73:807–14.

Endorsed by the American Academy of Pediatrics, Gidding SS, Dennison BA, et al. Dietary recommendations for children and adolescents: a guide for practitioners: consensus statement from the American Heart Association. Circulation 2005;112:2061–75.

Eskelinen MH, Ngandu T, Helkala E-L, et al. Fat intake at midlife and cognitive impairment later in life: a population-based CAIDE study. Int J Geriatr Psych 2008;23:741–7.

Esposito K, Giugliano D. Diet and inflammation: a link to metabolic and cardiovascular diseases. Eur Heart J 2006;27:15–20.

Fat. AHA Scientific Position. 2005. www.americanheart.org/presenter. jhtml?identifier=1582.

Fats and Cholesterol—The Good, the Bad, and the Healthy Diet. President and Fellows of Harvard College, 2006. www.hsph.harvard.edu/nutritionsource/fats.html.

Field AE, Willett WC, Lissner L, Colditz GA. Dietary fat and weight gain among women in the Nurses' Health Study. Obesity 2007;15:967–76.

Fish and Shellfish: Contamination Problems Preclude Inclusion in the Dietary Guidelines for Americans. Physicians Committee for Responsible Medicine, 2004. www.pcrm.org/health/reports/fish_report.html.

Forette F, Seux M-L, Staessen JA, et al. The prevention of dementia with antihypertensive treatment: new evidence from the Systolic Hypertension in Europe (Syst-Eur) study. [See comment.][Erratum appears in Arch Intern Med 2003 Jan 27;163(2):241.] Arch Intern Med 2002;162:2046–52.

Fratiglioni L, Paillard-Borg S, Winblad B. An active and socially integrated lifestyle in late life might protect against dementia. Lancet Neurology 2004;3:343–53.

Gesch CB, Hammond SM, Hampson SE, Eves A, Crowder MJ. Influence of supplementary vitamins, minerals and essential fatty acids on the antisocial behaviour of young adult prisoners: randomised, placebo-controlled trial. Brit J Psychiat 2002;181:22–8.

Ginsberg HN, Kris-Etherton P, Dennis B, et al. Effects of reducing dietary saturated fatty acids on plasma lipids and lipoproteins in healthy subjects: the Delta Study, Protocol 1. Arterioscl Throm Vas 1998;18:441–9.

Global Overfishing and International Fisheries Management. U.S. Senate Committee on Commerce, Science & Transportation, 2003. www.commerce.senate.gov/hearings/testimony.cfm?id=808&wit_id=2215.

Gomez-Pinilla F. Brain foods: the effects of nutrients on brain function. Nat Rev Neurosci 2008;9:568–78.

Gregg EW, Yaffe K, Cauley JA, et al. Is diabetes associated with cognitive impairment and cognitive decline among older women? Arch Intern Med 2000;160:174–80.

Griel AE, Kris-Etherton PM, Hilpert KF, Zhao G, West SG, Corwin RL. An increase in dietary n-3 fatty acids decreases a marker of bone resorption in humans. Nutr J 2007;6:2.

Guttman M. The aging brain. USC Health Magazine 2001 July 18.

Guyton AC, Hall JE. Textbook of Medical Physiology. 9th ed. Philadelphia: W. B. Saunders; 1996.

Hallahan B, Garland MR. Essential fatty acids and mental health. Brit J Psychiat 2005;186:275–7.

Hays NP, Starling RD, Liu X, et al. Effects of an ad libitum low-fat, high-carbohydrate diet on body weight, body composition, and fat distribution in older men and women: a randomized controlled trial. [See comment.] Arch Intern Med 2004;164:210–7.

Hu FB, Manson JE, Willett WC. Types of dietary fat and risk of coronary heart disease: a critical review. J Am Coll Nutr 2001;20:5–19.

Hu FB, Willett WC. Optimal diets for prevention of coronary heart disease. JAMA 2002;288:2569–78.

The Human Brain. The Franklin Institute Science Museum, The Franklin Institute Online, 2004. www.fi.edu/brain/index.htm.

Issa AM, Mojica WA, Morton SC, et al. The efficacy of omega-3 fatty acids on cognitive function in aging and dementia: a systematic review. Dement Geriatr Cogn 2006;21:88–96.

Jenab M, Ferrari P, Slimani N, et al. Association of nut and seed intake with colorectal cancer risk in the European Prospective Investigation into Cancer and Nutrition. Cancer Epidem Biomar 2004;13:1595–603.

Kang Jing X, Leaf A. Antiarrhythmic effects of polyunsaturated fatty acids: recent studies. Circulation 1996;94:1774–80.

Keeley J. Case Study: Appleton Central Alternative Charter High School's Nutrition and Wellness Program; 2004 December.

Keogh JB, Grieger JA, Noakes M, Clifton PM. Flow-mediated dilatation is impaired by a high-saturated fat diet but not by a high-carbohydrate diet. Arterioscl, Throm Vas 2005;25:1274–9.

Kivipelto M, Ngandu T, Fratiglioni L, et al. Obesity and vascular risk factors at midlife and the risk of dementia and Alzheimer disease. Arch Neurol 2005;62:1556–60.

Kris-Etherton PM. Monounsaturated fatty acids and risk of cardiovascular disease. Circulation 1999;100:1253–8.

Kris-Etherton P, Skulas Ann. Essential fatty acids and vegetarians: the missing link in long-chain omega-3 fatty acid recommendations. Nutrition & the MD 2005;31:1–4.

Kurzweil R. Live forever. Psychology Today 2000;33:66.

Kushi L, Giovannucci E. Dietary fat and cancer. Am J Med 2002;113 Suppl 9B:63S–70S.

Lewin MH, Bailey N, Bandaletova T, et al. Red meat enhances the colonic formation of the DNA adduct O6-carboxymethyl guanine: implications for colorectal cancer risk. Cancer Res 2006;66:1859–65.

Lindsay J, Laurin D, Verreault R, et al. Risk factors for Alzheimer's disease: a prospective analysis from the Canadian Study of Health and Aging. Am J Epidem 2002;156:445–53.

Lopez-Garcia E, Schulze MB, Manson JE, et al. Consumption of (n-3) fatty acids is related to plasma biomarkers of inflammation and endothelial activation in women. J Nutr 2004;134:1806–11.

MacLean CH, Mojica W, Morton SC, et al. Effects of omega-3 fatty acids on lipids and glycemic control in type II diabetes and the metabolic syndrome and on inflammatory bowel disease, rheumatoid arthritis, renal disease, systemic lupus erythematosus, and osteoporosis. In: AHRQ Publication No. 04-E012–2, ed. Evidence Report/ Technology Assessment: Agency for Healthcare Research and Quality. (Prepared by

Southern California/RAND Evidence-based Practice Center, under Contract No. 290-02-0003); 2004.

Mahaffey KR, Clickner RP, Bodurow CC. Blood organic mercury and dietary mercury intake: National Health and Nutrition Examination Survey, 1999 and 2000. [See comment.] Environ Health Persp 2004;112:562–70.

Marchioli R, Barzi F, Bomba E, et al. Early protection against sudden death by n-3 polyunsaturated fatty acids after myocardial infarction: time-course analysis of the results of the Gruppo Italiano per lo Studio della Sopravvivenza nell'Infarto Miocardico (GISSI)-Prevenzione. [See comment.] Circulation 2002;105:1897–903.

Matsuyama W, Mitsuyama H, Watanabe M, et al. Effects of omega-3 polyunsaturated fatty acids on inflammatory markers in COPD. [See comment.] Chest 2005;128:3817–27.

Mensink RP, Katan MB. Effect of dietary trans fatty acids on high-density and low-density lipoprotein cholesterol levels in healthy subjects. [See comment.] New Engl J Med 1990;323:439–45.

Merchant AT, Kelemen LE, de Koning L, et al. Interrelation of saturated fat, trans fat, alcohol intake, and subclinical atherosclerosis. Am J Clin Nutr 2008;87:168–74.

Morris MC, Evans DA, Bienias JL, et al. Dietary fats and the risk of incident Alzheimer disease. Arch Neurol 2003;60:194–200.

Morris MC, Evans DA, Bienias JL, Tangney CC, Wilson RS. Dietary fat intake and 6-year cognitive change in an older biracial community population. Neurology 2004;62:1573–9.

Morris MC, Evans DA, Tangney CC, Bienias JL, Wilson RS. Fish consumption and cognitive decline with age in a large community study. Arch Neurol 2005;62:1849–53.

Mosca L, Banka CL, Benjamin EJ, et al. Evidence-based guidelines for cardiovascular disease prevention in women: 2007 update. Circulation 2007; 115(11):1481–501.

Mozaffarian D. Trans fatty acids—effects on systemic inflammation and endothelial function. Atherosclerosis Supp 2006;7:29–32.

Mozaffarian D, Katan MB, Ascherio A, Stampfer MJ, Willett WC. Trans fatty acids and cardiovascular disease. New Engl J Med 2006;354:1601–13.

Mozaffarian D, Longstreth WT, Jr., Lemaitre RN, et al. Fish consumption and stroke risk in elderly individuals: the cardiovascular health study. [Erratum appears in Arch Intern Med. 2005 Mar 28;165(6):683.] Arch Intern Med 2005;165:200–6.

Mozaffarian D, Rimm EB. Fish intake, contaminants, and human health: evaluating the risks and the benefits. JAMA 2006;296:1885–99.

Mustad VA, Etherton TD, Cooper AD, et al. Reducing saturated fat intake is associated with increased levels of LDL receptors on mononuclear cells in healthy men and women. J Lipid Res 1997;38:459–68.

My Pyramid.Gov. Why Is It Important to Make Lean or Low-Fat Choices from the Meat and Beans Group? U.S. Department of Agriculture, 2005. www.mypyramid.gov/pyramid/meat_why_print.html.

Nash DT, Fillit H. Cardiovascular disease risk factors and cognitive impairment. Am J Cardiol 2006;97:1262–5.

National Cholesterol Education Program. ATP III Guidelines At-A-Glance. Quick Desk Reference. Reference: U.S. Department of Health and Human Services. Public

Health Service. National Institutes of Health. National Heart, Lung, and Blood Institute; 2001 May. Report No.: 01-3305.

Nemets H, Nemets B, Apter A, Bracha Z, Belmaker RH. Omega-3 treatment of childhood depression: a controlled, double-blind pilot study. Am J Psychiat 2006;163:1098–100.

Newman AB, Fitzpatrick AL, Lopez O, et al. Dementia and Alzheimer's disease incidence in relationship to cardiovascular disease in the cardiovascular health study cohort. J Am Geriatr Soc 2005;53:1101–7.

Ngandu T, von Strauss E, Helkala EL, et al. Education and dementia: What lies behind the association? Neurology 2007;69:1442–50.

Nicholls SJ, Lundman P, Harmer JA, et al. Consumption of saturated fat impairs the anti-inflammatory properties of high-density lipoproteins and endothelial function. J Am Coll Cardiol 2006;48:715–20.

Norat T, Bingham S, Ferrari P, et al. Meat, fish, and colorectal cancer risk: The European Prospective Investigation into Cancer and Nutrition. J Natl Cancer I 2005;97:906–16.

Oh K, Hu FB, Manson JE, Stampfer MJ, Willett WC. Dietary fat intake and risk of coronary heart disease in women: 20 years of follow-up of the Nurses' Health Study. Am J Epidem 2005;161:672–9.

Oh R. Practical applications of fish oil ({omega}-3 fatty acids) in primary care. J Am Board Fam Pract 2005;18:28–36.

Omega-3 Fatty Acids and Health. 2005. www.dietary-supplements.info.nih.gov/ FactSheets/Omega3FattyAcidsandHealth.asp.

Panza F, Solfrizzi V, Colacicco AM, et al. Mediterranean diet and cognitive decline. Public Health Nutr 2004;7:959–63.

Pappolla MA, Bryant-Thomas TK, Herbert D, et al. Mild hypercholesterolemia is an early risk factor for the development of Alzheimer amyloid pathology. Neurology 2003;61:199–205.

Peet M, Laugharne JDE, Mellor J, Ramchand CN. Essential fatty acid deficiency in erythrocyte membranes from chronic schizophrenic patients, and the clinical effects of dietary supplementation. Prostag Leukotr Ess 1996;55:71–5.

Pirro M, Schillaci G, Savarese G, et al. Attenutation of inflammation with short-term dietary intervention is associated with a reduction of arterial stiffness in subjects with hypercholesterolaemia. Eur J Cardiov Prev R 2004;11:497–502.

Siegel GJ, Agranoff BW, Fisher SK, Albers RW, Uhler MD, eds. Basic Neurochemistry: Molecular, Cellular and Medical Aspects. 6th ed. Philadelphia: American Society for Neurochemistry, Lippincott Williams and Wilkins; 1999. www.ncbi.nlm.nih.gov/ books/bv.fcgi?rid=bnchm; 1999.

Simopoulos AP. Evolutionary aspects of diet, the omega-6/omega-3 ratio and genetic variation: nutritional implications for chronic diseases. Biomed Pharmacother 2006;60:502–7.

Sinha R, Cross AJ, Graubard BI, Leitzmann MF, Schatzkin A. Meat intake and mortality: a prospective study of over half a million people. Arch Intern Med 2009;169:562–71.

Solfrizzi V, Colacicco AM, D'Introno A, et al. Dietary intake of unsaturated fatty acids and age-related cognitive decline: a 8.5-year follow-up of the Italian Longitudinal Study on Aging. Neurobiol Aging 2006;27:1694–704.

Solfrizzi V, D'Introno A, Colacicco AM, et al. Dietary fatty acids intake: possible role in cognitive decline and dementia. Exp Gerontol 2005;40:257–70.

Solfrizzi V, Panza F, Torres F, et al. High monounsaturated fatty acids intake protects against age-related cognitive decline. Neurology 1999;52:1563–9.

Stampfer MJ. Cardiovascular disease and Alzheimer's disease: common links. J Intern Med 2006;260:211–23.

Su K-P, Huang S-Y, Chiu C-C, Shen WW. Omega-3 fatty acids in major depressive disorder: a preliminary double-blind, placebo-controlled trial. Eur Neuropsychopharm 2003;13:267–71.

Sublette ME, Hibbeln JR, Galfalvy H, Oquendo MA, Mann JJ. Omega-3 polyunsaturated essential fatty acid status as a predictor of future suicide risk. Am J Psychiat 2006;163:1100–2.

Sung J, DeRegis JR, Bacher AC, et al. Lower dietary polyunsaturated to saturated fat ratio is associated with increased visceral adiposity. In: American College of Cardiology Annual Meeting, Lipids—Clinical and Prevention; 2003 March 30; Chicago. Abstract; 2003. p. Abstract.

Temme EH, Mensink RP, Hornstra G. Comparison of the effects of diets enriched in lauric, palmitic, or oleic acids on serum lipids and lipoproteins in healthy women and men. Am J Clin Nutr 1996;63:897–903.

Uauy R, Dangour AD. Nutrition in brain development and aging: role of essential fatty acids nutrition in brain development and aging. role of essential fatty acids. Nutr Rev 2006;64:S24–S33.

USDA National Nutrient Database for Standard Reference. Release 18. United States Department of Agriculture. Agricultural Research Service, 2005. www.nal.usda.gov/fnic/foodcomp/Data/SR18/sr18.html.

U.S. Department of Health and Human Services, National Institutes of Health, National Institute on Aging. Progress Report on Alzheimer's Disease 2004–2005: National Institutes of Health; 2005 November. Report No.: NIH publication 05-5724.

Wang L, Folsom AR, Zheng Z-J, Pankow JS, Eckfeldt JH. Plasma fatty acid composition and incidence of diabetes in middle-aged adults: the Atherosclerosis Risk in Communities (ARIC) Study. Am J Clin Nutr 2003;78:91–8.

Willett WC. Ask the doctor. I have heard that coconut is bad for the heart and that it is good for the heart. Which is right? Harvard Heart Letter 2006;17:8.

Willet WC, Ascherio A. Trans fatty acids: are the effects only marginal? Am J Public Health 1994;sect. 722–4.

Yaffe K, Blackwell T, Kanaya AM, Davidowitz N, Barrett-Connor E, Krueger K. Diabetes, impaired fasting glucose, and development of cognitive impairment in older women. Neurology 2004;63:658–63.

Yaffe K, Kanaya A, Lindquist K, et al. The metabolic syndrome, inflammation, and risk of cognitive decline. JAMA 2004;292:2237–42.

Yu-Poth S, Etherton TD, Reddy CC, et al. Lowering dietary saturated fat and total fat reduces the oxidative susceptibility of LDL in healthy men and women. J Nutr 2000;130:2228–37.

Zhang J, Hebert JR, Muldoon MF. Dietary fat intake is associated with psychosocial and cognitive functioning of school-aged children in the United States. J Nutr 2005;135:1967–73.

## Chapter 2

Akbaraly NT, Hininger-Favier I, Carriere I, et al. Plasma selenium over time and cognitive decline in the elderly. Epidemiology 2007;18:52–8.

American Heart Association, American Stroke Association. Heart Disease and Stroke Statistics—2008 Update. Our Guide to Current Statistics and the Supplement to Our Heart and Stroke Facts. Dallas: American Heart Association, American Stroke Association; 2008.

Appel LJ, Sacks FM, Carey VJ, et al. Effects of protein, monounsaturated fat, and carbohydrate intake on blood pressure and serum lipids: results of the OmniHeart Randomized Trial. JAMA 2005;294:2455–64.

Bazzano LA, He J, Ogden LG, et al. Legume consumption and risk of coronary heart disease in US men and women: NHANES I Epidemiologic Follow-up Study. [See comment.] Arch Intern Med 2001;161:2573–8.

Berr C, Balansard B, Arnaud J, Roussel AM, Alperovitch A. Cognitive decline is associated with systemic oxidative stress: the EVA study. Etude du Vieillissement Arteriel. J Am Geriatr Soc 2000;48:1285–91.

Bopp MJ, Houston DK, Lenchik L, Easter L, Kritchevsky SB, Nicklas BJ. Lean mass loss is associated with low protein intake during dietary-induced weight loss in postmenopausal women. J Am Diet Assoc 2008;108:1216–20.

Cai H, Shu XO, Gao Y-T, Li H, Yang G, Zheng W. A prospective study of dietary patterns and mortality in Chinese women. Epidemiology 2007;18:393–401.

Cho E, Chen WY, Hunter DJ, et al. Red meat intake and risk of breast cancer among premenopausal women. Arch Intern Med 2006;166:2253–9.

Committee on Military Nutrition Research, Institute of Medicine. The Role of Protein and Amino Acids in Sustaining and Enhancing Performance. Washington, DC: National Academy Press; 1999.

Cross AJ, Leitzmann MF, Gail MH, Hollenbeck AR, Schatzkin A, Sinha R. A prospective study of red and processed meat intake in relation to cancer risk. PLoS Med 2007;4:e325.

Cui X, Dai Q, Tseng M, Shu X-O, Gao Y-T, Zheng W. Dietary patterns and breast cancer risk in the Shanghai Breast Cancer Study. Cancer Epidem Biomar 2007;16:1443–8.

Dietary Supplement Fact Sheet: Selenium. Office of Dietary Supplements, National Institutes of Health, 2004. www.ods.od.nih.gov/factsheets/selenium.asp#h2.

Elliott P, Stamler J, Dyer AR, et al. Association between protein intake and blood pressure: The INTERMAP study. Arch Intern Med 2006;166:79–87.

Embassy of the United States, Jakarta Indonesia. Indonesia: Environment, science, and technology, and health highlights January/February 2005. In: Recent Economic Reports: American Embassy Information Resource Center; 2006.

Epel E, Jimenez S, Brownell K, Stroud L, Stoney C, Niaura R. Are stress eaters at risk for the metabolic syndrome? Ann NY Acad Sci 2004;1032:208–10.

Epel E, Lapidus R, McEwen B, Brownell K. Stress may add bite to appetite in women: a laboratory study of stress-induced cortisol and eating behavior. Psychoneuroendocrinology 2001;26:37–49.

Fernstrom JD. The influence of dietary protein and amino acids on brain function. Trends Food Sci Tech 1991;2:201–4.

Franco OH, Burger H, Lebrun CEI, et al. Higher dietary intake of lignans is associated with better cognitive performance in postmenopausal women. J Nutr 2005;135:1190–5.

Fulgoni VL, III. Current protein intake in America: analysis of the National Health and Nutrition Examination Survey, 2003–2004. Am J Clin Nutr 2008;87:1554S–7.

Fung T, Hu FB, Fuchs C, et al. Major dietary patterns and the risk of colorectal cancer in women. Arch Intern Med 2003;163:309–14.

Fung TT, Schulze M, Manson JE, Willett WC, Hu FB. Dietary patterns, meat intake, and the risk of type 2 diabetes in women. Arch Intern Med 2004;164:2235–40.

Gaine PC, Pikosky MA, Martin WF, Bolster DR, Maresh CM, Rodriguez NR. Level of dietary protein impacts whole body protein turnover in trained males at rest. Metabolism 2006;55:501–7.

Gao S, Jin Y, Hall KS, et al. Selenium level and cognitive function in rural elderly Chinese. Am J Epidem 2007;165:955–65.

Giovannucci E, Rimm EB, Stampfer MJ, Colditz GA, Ascherio A, Willett WC. Intake of fat, meat, and fiber in relation to risk of colon cancer in men. Cancer Res 1994;54:2390–7.

Guo C, Wilkens LR, Maskarinec G, et al. Examining associations of brain aging with midlife tofu consumption. J Am Coll Nutr 2000;19:467–8.

Halford JCG, Harrold JA, Boyland EJ, Lawton CL, Blundell JE. Serotonergic drugs: effects on appetite expression and use for the treatment of obesity. Drugs 2007;67:27–55.

Halton TL, Hu FB. The effects of high protein diets on thermogenesis, satiety and weight loss: a critical review. J Am Coll Nutr 2004;23:373–85.

Henkel J. Soy: health claims for soy protein, questions about other components: U.S. Food and Drug Administration, FDA Consumer; 2000 May–June.

Hogervorst E, Sadjimim T, Yesufu A, Kreager P, Rahardjo TB. High tofu intake is associated with worse memory in elderly Indonesian men and women. Dement Geriatr Cogn 2008;26:50–7.

Hu FB, Rimm EB, Stampfer MJ, Ascherio A, Spiegelman D, Willett WC. Prospective study of major dietary patterns and risk of coronary heart disease in men. Am J Clin Nutr 2000;72:912–21.

Hu FB, Stampfer MJ, Manson JE, et al. Frequent nut consumption and risk of coronary heart disease in women: prospective cohort study. [See comment.] Brit Med J 1998;317:1341–5.

Hunt SM, Groff JL. Advanced Nutrition and Human Metabolism. St. Paul: West Publishing Co.; 1990.

Hymowitz T, Shurtleff WR. Debunking soybean myths and legends in the historical and popular literature. Crop Sci 2005;45:473–6.

Iglay HB, Thyfault JP, Apolzan JW, Campbell WW. Resistance training and dietary protein: effects on glucose tolerance and contents of skeletal muscle insulin signaling proteins in older persons. Am J Clin Nutr 2007;85:1005–13.

Institute of Medicine. Dietary reference intakes: water, potassium, sodium, chloride, and sulfate. Washington, DC: National Academies Press; 2004.

Jenab M, Ferrari P, Slimani N, et al. Association of nut and seed intake with colorectal cancer risk in the European Prospective Investigation into Cancer and Nutrition. Cancer Epidem Biomar 2004;13:1595–603.

Jiang R, Jacobs DR, Jr., Mayer-Davis E, et al. Nut and seed consumption and inflammatory markers in the multi-ethnic study of atherosclerosis. Am J Epidem 2006;163:222–31.

Jiang R, Manson JE, Stamfer MJ, Simin L, Willett WC, Hu FB. Nut and peanut butter consumption and risk of type 2 diabetes in women. JAMA 2002;288:2554–60.

Kelly JH, Jr., Sabate J. Nuts and coronary heart disease: an epidemiological perspective. Brit J Nutr 2006;96:S61–S7.

Kessler DA. The End of Overeating: Taking Control of the Insatiable American Appetite. New York: Rodale; 2009.

Kokubo Y, Iso H, Ishihara J, et al. Association of dietary intake of soy, beans, and isoflavones with risk of cerebral and myocardial infarctions in Japanese populations: the Japan Public Health Center-based (JPHC) study cohort I. Circulation 2007;116:2553–62.

Kulisevsky J. Role of dopamine in learning and memory: implications for the treatment of cognitive dysfunction in patients with Parkinson's disease. Drugs Aging 2000;16:365–79.

Kurzweil R. Live forever. Psychology Today 2000;33:66.

Lanza E, Hartman TJ, Albert PS, et al. High dry bean intake and reduced risk of advanced colorectal adenoma recurrence among participants in the polyp prevention trial. J Nutr 2006;136:1896–903.

Lemon PWR. Beyond the zone: protein needs of active individuals. J Am Coll Nutr 2000;19:513S-21.

Marangoni F, Colombo C, Martiello A, Poli A, Paoletti R, Galli C. Levels of the n-3 fatty acid eicosapentaenoic acid in addition to those of alpha linolenic acid are significantly raised in blood lipids by the intake of four walnuts a day in humans. Nutr Metab Cardiovas 2007;17:457–61.

McEwen BS. Protection and damage from acute and chronic stress: allostasis and allostatic overload and relevance to the pathophysiology of psychiatric disorders. Ann NY Acad Sci 2004;1032:1–7.

McGee H. On Food and Cooking: The Science and Lore of the Kitchen. New York: Charles Scribner's Sons; 1984.

Meck WH, Williams CL. Metabolic imprinting of choline by its availability during gestation: implications for memory and attentional processing across the lifespan. Neurosci Biobehav R 2003;27:385–99.

Merchant AT, Anand SS, Vuksan V, et al. Protein intake is inversely associated with abdominal obesity in a multi-ethnic population. J Nutr 2005;135:1196–201.

Messina M, Messina V. Provisional recommended soy protein and isoflavone intakes for healthy adults: rationale. (Food Science). Nutrition Today 2003;38:100(10).

Michels KB, Giovannucci E, Chan AT, Singhania R, Fuchs CS, Willett WC. Fruit and vegetable consumption and colorectal adenomas in the Nurses' Health Study. Cancer Res 2006;66:3942–53.

O'Connor DB, Jones F, Conner M, McMillan B, Ferguson E. Effects of daily hassles and eating style on eating behavior. Health Psychol 2008;27:S20–31.

Paddon-Jones D, Short KR, Campbell WW, Volpi E, Wolfe RR. Role of dietary protein in the sarcopenia of aging. Am J Clin Nutr 2008;87:1562S–6.

Paddon-Jones D, Westman E, Mattes RD, Wolfe RR, Astrup A, Westerterp-Plantenga M. Protein, weight management, and satiety. Am J Clin Nutr 2008;87:1558S–61.

Patel G. Essential fats in walnuts are good for the heart and diabetes. J Am Diet Assoc 2005;105:1096–7.

Piggott MA, Ballard CG, Rowan E, et al. Selective loss of dopamine D2 receptors in temporal cortex in dementia with Lewy bodies, association with cognitive decline. Synapse 2007;61:903–11.

Ros E, Nunez I, Perez-Heras A, et al. A walnut diet improves endothelial function in hypercholesterolemic subjects: a randomized crossover trial. Circulation 2004;109:1609–14.

Sacks FM, Lichtenstein A, Van Horn L, et al. Soy protein, isoflavones, and cardiovascular health: an American Heart Association science advisory for professionals from the Nutrition Committee. Circulation 2006;113:1034–44.

Schliebs R, Arendt T. The significance of the cholinergic system in the brain during aging and in Alzheimer's disease. J Neural Transm 2006;113:1625–44.

Shai I, Schwarzfuchs D, Henkin Y, et al. Weight loss with a low-carbohydrate, Mediterranean, or low-fat diet. New Engl J Med 2008;359:229–41.

Siegel GJ, Agranoff BW, Fisher SK, Albers RW, Uhler MD, eds. Basic Neurochemistry Molecular, Cellular and Medical Aspects. 6th ed. Philadelphia: Lippincott Williams and Wilkins. Copyright by American Society for Neurochemistry. www.ncbi.nlm. nih.gov/books/bv.fcgi?rid=bnchm; 1999.

Soybeans: The Success Story. National Soybean Research Laboratory, University of Illinois Urbana-Champaign, 2008. www.nsrl.uiuc.edu/aboutsoy/history1.html.

Soy Stats 2008. The American Soybean Association, 2008. www.soystats.com/2008/Default-frames.htm.

Szeszko PR, Betensky JD, Mentschel C, et al. Increased stress and smaller anterior hippocampal volume. Neuroreport 2006;17:1825–8.

Torres SJ, Nowson CA. Relationship between stress, eating behavior, and obesity. Nutrition 2007;23:887–94.

Ueshima H, Stamler J, Elliott P, et al. Food omega-3 fatty acid intake of individuals (total, linolenic acid, long-chain) and their blood pressure: INTERMAP study. Hypertension 2007;50:313–9.

United Soybean Board. www.soybean.org.

USDA National Nutrient Database for Standard Reference. Release 20. U.S. Department of Agriculture. Agricultural Research Service, 2007. www.ars.usda.gov/ba/bhnrc/ndl.

Varraso R, Fung TT, Barr RG, Hu FB, Willett W, Camargo CA, Jr. Prospective study of dietary patterns and chronic obstructive pulmonary disease among US women. Am J Clin Nutr 2007;86:488–95.

Villegas R, Gao Y-T, Yang G, et al. Legume and soy food intake and the incidence of type 2 diabetes in the Shanghai Women's Health Study. Am J Clin Nutr 2008;87:162–7.

White LR, Petrovitch H, Ross GW, et al. Brain aging and midlife tofu consumption. J Am Coll Nutr 2000;19:242–55.

Whitney EN HE, Rolfes SR. Understanding Nutrition. St. Paul: West Publishing Co.;
    1990.
Wien MA, Sabate JM, Ikle DN, Cole SE, Kandeel FR. Almonds vs complex carbo-
    hydrates in a weight reduction program. [Erratum appears in Int J Obes Relat
    Metab Disord 2004 Mar;28(3):459.] Int J Obes Relat Metab Disord, Journal of the
    International Association for the Study of Obesity 2003;27:1365–72.
Willett W. Eat, Drink and Be Healthy: The Harvard Medical School Guide to Healthy
    Eating. New York: Simon & Schuster; 2001.
Williams M. Dietary supplements and sports performance: amino acids. (Commentary)
    Journal of the International Society of Sports Nutrition 2005;2:63(5).
Williams RW, Herrup K. The control of neuron number. In: The Annual Review of
    Neuroscience; 1988, 423–53. Revised September 28, 2001.
Wurtman JJ. Depression and weight gain: the serotonin connection. J Affect Disorders
    1993;29:183–92.
Yang G, Shu X-O, Jin F, et al. Longitudinal study of soy food intake and blood pressure
    among middle-aged and elderly Chinese women. Am J Clin Nutr 2005;81:1012–7.
Zeisel SH. Nutritional importance of choline for brain development. J Am Coll Nutr
    2004;23:621S–6.
Zeisel SH, Blusztajn JK. Choline and human nutrition. Ann Rev of Nutr 1994;14:269–96.
Zhang X, Shu XO, Gao Y-T, et al. Soy food consumption is associated with lower risk of
    coronary heart disease in Chinese women. J Nutr 2003;133:2874–8.
Zhao G, Etherton TD, Martin KR, West SG, Gillies PJ, Kris-Etherton PM. Dietary
    {alpha}-linolenic acid reduces inflammatory and lipid cardiovascular risk factors in
    hypercholesterolemic men and women. J Nutr 2004;134:2991–7.
Zhou J-R. Soy and the prevention of lifestyle-related diseases. Clin Exp Pharmacol P
    2004;31:S14–S9.

## Chapter 3

Agudo A, Cabrera L, Amiano P, et al. Fruit and vegetable intakes, dietary antioxidant
    nutrients, and total mortality in Spanish adults: findings from the Spanish cohort of
    the European Prospective Investigation into Cancer and Nutrition (EPIC-Spain). Am
    J Clin Nutr 2007;85:1634–42.
Angus M, Brown BRR. Astrocyte glycogen and brain energy metabolism. Glia
    2007;55:1263–71.
Barberger-Gateau P, Letenneur L, Deschamps V, Peres K, Dartigues J-F, Renaud S. Fish,
    meat, and risk of dementia: cohort study. Brit Med J 2002;325:932–3.
Barnard ND, Cohen J, Jenkins DJA, et al. A low-fat vegan diet improves glycemic control
    and cardiovascular risk factors in a randomized clinical trial in individuals with type
    2 diabetes. Diabetes Care 2006;29:1777–83.
Bassuk SS, Manson JE. Lifestyle and risk of cardiovascular disease and type 2 diabetes
    in women: a review of the epidemiologic evidence. American Journal of Lifestyle
    Medicine 2008;2:191–213.
Behall KM, Scholfield DJ, Hallfrisch J. Whole-grain diets reduce blood pressure in
    mildly hypercholesterolemic men and women. J Am Diet Assoc 2006;106:1445–9.

Block G. Foods contributing to energy intake in the US: data from NHANES III and NHANES 1999–2000. J Food Compos Anal 2004;17:439–47.

Brand-Miller JC. Glycemic load and chronic disease. Nutr Rev 2003;61:S49–55.

Bray GA, Nielsen SJ, Popkin BM. Consumption of high-fructose corn syrup in beverages may play a role in the epidemic of obesity. [See comment.] [Erratum appears in Am J Clin Nutr 2004 Oct;80(4):1090.] Am J Clin Nutr 2004;79:537–43.

Butterfield DA, Reed T, Newman SF, Sultana R. Roles of amyloid [beta]-peptide-associated oxidative stress and brain protein modifications in the pathogenesis of Alzheimer's disease and mild cognitive impairment. Free Radical Bio Med 2007;43:658–77.

Centers for Disease Control and Prevention. Fruit and vegetable consumption among adults—United States, 2005. In: MMWR, Morb Mortal Wkly Rep 56(10);213–217; 2007.

Centers for Disease Control and Prevention. Number of people with diabetes increases to 24 million. Washington, DC: Department of Health & Human Services; 2008. www.cdc.gov/media/pressrel/2008/r080624.htm.

Davies MJ, Judd JT, Baer DJ, et al. Black tea consumption reduces total and LDL cholesterol in mildly hypercholesterolemic adults. J Nutr 2003;133;3298S–302S.

Drachman DA. Aging of the brain, entropy, and Alzheimer disease. Neurology 2006;67:1340–52.

Droge W, Schipper HM. Oxidative stress and aberrant signaling in aging and cognitive decline. Aging Cell 2007;6:361–70.

Du H, van der A DL, van Bakel MME, et al. Glycemic index and glycemic load in relation to food and nutrient intake and metabolic risk factors in a Dutch population. Am J Clin Nutr 2008;87:655–61.

Fung TT, Hu FB, Pereira MA, et al. Whole-grain intake and the risk of type 2 diabetes: a prospective study in men. Am J Clin Nutr 2002;76:535–40.

Fung TT, Malik V, Rexrode KM, Manson JE, Willett WC, Hu FB. Sweetened beverage consumption and risk of coronary heart disease in women. Am J Clin Nutr 2009;89:1037–42.

Fung TT, Willett WC, Stampfer MJ, Manson JE, Hu FB. Dietary patterns and the risk of coronary heart disease in women. Arch Intern Med 2001;161:1857–62.

Gardner CD, Coulston A, Chatterjee L, Rigby A, Spiller G, Farquhar JW. The effect of a plant-based diet on plasma lipids in hypercholesterolemic adults: a randomized trial. [See comment.] [Summary for patients in Ann Intern Med 2005 May 3;142(9):I35; PMID: 15867398.] Ann Intern Med 2005;142:725–33.

Greenwood CE. Dietary carbohydrate, glucose regulation, and cognitive performance in elderly persons. Nutr Rev 2003;61:S68–74.

Greenwood CE, Kaplan RJ, Hebblethwaite S, Jenkins DJA. Carbohydrate-induced memory impairment in adults with type 2 diabetes. Diabetes Care 2003;26:1961–6.

Gregg EW, Yaffe K, Cauley JA, et al. Is diabetes associated with cognitive impairment and cognitive decline among older women? Arch Intern Med 2000;160:174–80.

Gross LS, Li L, Ford ES, Liu S. Increased consumption of refined carbohydrates and the epidemic of type 2 diabetes in the United States: an ecologic assessment. [See comment.] Am J Clin Nutr 2004;79:774–9.

Harding A-H, Wareham NJ, Bingham SA, et al. Plasma vitamin C level, fruit and vegetable consumption, and the risk of new-onset type 2 diabetes mellitus: The European Prospective Investigation of Cancer-Norfolk Prospective Study. Arch Intern Med 2008;168:1493–9.

Hirani V, Zaninotto P, Primatesta P. Generalised and abdominal obesity and risk of diabetes, hypertension and hypertension-diabetes co-morbidity in England. Public Health Nutr 2008;11:521–7.

Hu FB. Plant-based foods and prevention of cardiovascular disease: an overview. Am J Clin Nutr 2003;78:544S-51.

Hu FB, Willett WC. Optimal diets for prevention of coronary heart disease. JAMA 2002 288:2569–78.

Jacobs DR, Jr., Andersen LF, Blomhoff R. Whole-grain consumption is associated with a reduced risk of noncardiovascular, noncancer death attributed to inflammatory diseases in the Iowa Women's Health Study. Am J Clin Nutr 2007;85:1606–14.

Kang JH, Ascherio A, Grodstein F. Fruit and vegetable consumption and cognitive decline in aging women. Ann Neurol 2005;57:713–20.

Kaplan RJ, Greenwood CE, Winocur G, Wolever TMS. Cognitive performance is associated with glucose regulation in healthy elderly persons and can be enhanced with glucose and dietary carbohydrates. Am J Clin Nutr 2000;72:825–36.

Kaplan RJ, Greenwood CE, Winocur G, Wolever TMS. Dietary protein, carbohydrate, and fat enhance memory performance in the healthy elderly. Am J Clin Nutr 2001;74:687–93.

Kodl CT, Seaquist ER. Cognitive dysfunction and diabetes mellitus. Endocr Rev 2008;29:494–511.

Korol DL, Gold PE. Glucose, memory, and aging. Am J Clin Nutr 1998;67:764S-71.

Krishnan S, Rosenberg L, Singer M, et al. Glycemic index, glycemic load, and cereal fiber intake and risk of type 2 diabetes in US black women. Arch Intern Med 2007;167:2304–9.

Kuriyama S, Hozawa A, Ohmori K, et al. Green tea consumption and cognitive function: a cross-sectional study from the Tsurugaya Project 1. Am J Clin Nutr 2006;83:355–61.

Kuriyama S, Shimazu T, Ohmori K, et al. Green tea consumption and mortality due to cardiovascular disease, cancer, and all causes in Japan: the Ohsaki study. JAMA 2006;296:1255–65.

Lieberman HR, Falco CM, Slade SS. Carbohydrate administration during a day of sustained aerobic activity improves vigilance, as assessed by a novel ambulatory monitoring device, and mood. Am J Clin Nutr 2002;76:120–7.

Liu S. Intake of refined carbohydrates and whole grain foods in relation to risk of type 2 diabetes mellitus and coronary heart disease. J Am Coll Nutr 2002;21:298–306.

Liu S, Manson JE, Buring JE, Stampfer MJ, Willett WC, Ridker PM. Relation between a diet with a high glycemic load and plasma concentrations of high-sensitivity C-reactive protein in middle-aged women. Am J Clin Nutr 2002;75:492–8.

Liu S, Manson JE, Stampfer MJ, et al. Whole grain consumption and risk of ischemic stroke in women: a prospective study. JAMA 2000;284:1534–40.

Liu S, Stampfer MJ, Hu FB, et al. Whole-grain consumption and risk of coronary heart disease: results from the Nurses' Health Study. Am J Clin Nutr 1999;70:412–9.

Lovell, MA. WRM. Oxidative damage in mild cognitive impairment and early
    Alzheimer's disease. J Neurosci Res 2007;85:3036–40.

Lutsey PL, Steffen LM, Stevens J. Dietary intake and the development of the metabolic
    syndrome: The Atherosclerosis Risk in Communities Study. [Article.] Circulation
    2008;117:754–61.

Malik VS, Willett WC, Hu FB. Sugar-sweetened beverages and BMI in children and
    adolescents: reanalyses of a meta-analysis. Am J Clin Nutr 2009;89:438–9.

McGee H. On Food and Cooking: The Science and Lore of the Kitchen. New York:
    Charles Scribner's Sons; 1984.

McKeown NM, Meigs JB, Liu S, Wilson PWF, Jacques PF. Whole-grain intake is
    favorably associated with metabolic risk factors for type 2 diabetes and cardiovascular
    disease in the Framingham Offspring Study. Am J Clin Nutr 2002;76:390–8.

Molan PC. Potential of honey in the treatment of wounds and burns. Am J Clin
    Dermatol 2001;2:13–9.

Murakami K, Sasaki S, Okubo H, Takahashi Y, Hosoi Y, Itabashi M. Dietary fiber
    intake, dietary glycemic index and load, and body mass index: a cross-sectional study
    of 3931 Japanese women aged 18–20 years. Eur J Clin Nutr 2007;61:986–95.

Nanri A, Mizoue T, Yoshida D, Takahashi R, Takayanagi R. Dietary patterns and A1C
    in Japanese men and women. Diabetes Care 2008;31:1568–73.

National Center for Chronic Disease Prevention and Health Promotion. PreDiabetes.
    Frequently Asked Questions. Diabetes Public Health Resource 2007.

National Cholesterol Education Program, Third Report of the Expert Panel on
    Detection, Evaluation, and Treatment of High Blood Cholesterol in Adults (Adult
    Treatment Panel III), National Heart, Lung, and Blood Institute, National Institutes
    of Health, May 2001.

National Diabetes Information Clearinghouse. National Diabetes Statistics, 2007. In:
    NIH Publication No 08-3892. June 2008 ed: National Institute of Diabetes and
    Digestive and Kidney Diseases, National Institutes of Health; 2007.

Newby PK. Plant based diet may help control weight. Agricultural Research Magazine,
    U.S. Department of Agriculture 2006;54.

Ng T-P, Feng L, Niti M, Kua E-H, Yap K-B. Tea consumption and cognitive impairment
    and decline in older Chinese adults. Am J Clin Nutr 2008;88:224–31.

Nothlings U, Schulze MB, Weikert C, et al. Intake of vegetables, legumes, and fruit,
    and risk for all-cause, cardiovascular, and cancer mortality in a European diabetic
    population. J Nutr 2008;138:775–81.

Palmer JR, Boggs DA, Krishnan S, Hu FB, Singer M, Rosenberg L. Sugar-sweetened
    beverages and incidence of type 2 diabetes mellitus in African American women.
    Arch Intern Med 2008;168:1487–92.

Rana JS, Li TY, Manson JE, Hu FB. Adiposity compared with physical inactivity and
    risk of type 2 diabetes in women. Diabetes Care 2007;30:53–8.

Sahyoun NR, Jacques PF, Zhang XL, Juan W, McKeown NM. Whole-grain intake is
    inversely associated with the metabolic syndrome and mortality in older adults. Am J
    Clin Nutr 2006;83:124–31.

Salmeron J, Manson JE, Stampfer MJ, Colditz GA, Wing AL, Willett WC. Dietary
    fiber, glycemic load, and risk of non-insulin-dependent diabetes mellitus in women.
    [See comment]. JAMA 1997;277:472–7.

Schramm DD, Karim M, Schrader HR, Holt RR, Cardetti M, Keen CL. Honey with high levels of antioxidants can provide protection to healthy human subjects. J Agr Food Chem 2003;51:1732–5.

Schulze MB, Manson JE, Ludwig DS, et al. Sugar-sweetened beverages, weight gain, and incidence of type 2 diabetes in young and middle-aged women. [See comment.] JAMA 2004;292:927–34.

Seely D, Mills EJ, Wu P, Verma S, Guyatt GH. The effects of green tea consumption on incidence of breast cancer and recurrence of breast cancer: a systematic review and meta-analysis. Integr Cancer Ther 2005;4:144–55.

Siegel GJ, Agranoff BW, Fisher SK, Albers RW, Uhler MD, eds. Basic Neurochemistry Molecular, Cellular and Medical Aspects. 6th ed. Philadelphia: Lippincott Williams and Wilkins. Copyright by American Society for Neurochemistry. www.ncbi.nlm.nih.gov/books/bv.fcgi?rid=bnchm; 1999.

Sommerfield AJ, Deary IJ, Frier BM. Acute hyperglycemia alters mood state and impairs cognitive performance in people with type 2 diabetes. Diabetes Care 2004;27:2335–40.

Stanhope KL. Consuming fructose-sweetened, not glucose-sweetened, beverages increases visceral adiposity and lipids and decreases insulin sensitivity in overweight/obese humans. J Clin Invest 2009;119:1322–34.

Sueoka N, Suganuma M, Sueoka E, et al. A new function of green tea: prevention of lifestyle-related diseases. Ann NY Acad Sci 2001;928:274–80.

Thomas DE, Elliott EJ, Baur L. Low glycaemic index or low glycaemic load diets for overweight and obesity. Cochrane Db Syst Rev 2007:CD005105.

U.S. Department of Health and Human Services, National Institutes of Health, National Heart Lung and Blood Institute. Your guide to lowering your blood pressure with DASH. In: DASH Eating Plan Lower Your Blood Pressure, NIH Publication No 06–4082 U.S. Department of Health and Human Services; 2006.

Villegas R, Liu S, Gao Y-T, et al. Prospective study of dietary carbohydrates, glycemic index, glycemic load, and incidence of type 2 diabetes mellitus in middle-aged Chinese women. Arch Intern Med 2007;167:2310–6.

Vos MB, Kimmons JE, Gillespie C, Welsh J, Blanck HM. Dietary fructose consumption among US children and adults: the Third National Health and Nutrition Examination Survey. [See comment.] Medscape Journal of Medicine 2008;10:160.

Wang L, Gaziano JM, Liu S, Manson JE, Buring JE, Sesso HD. Whole- and refined-grain intakes and the risk of hypertension in women. Am J Clin Nutr 2007;86:472–9.

Whitney EN HE, Rolfes SR. Understanding Nutrition. St. Paul: West Publishing Co.; 1990.

Willett W. Eat, Drink and Be Healthy: The Harvard Medical School Guide to Healthy Eating. New York: Simon & Schuster; 2001.

Willett W, Manson J, Liu S. Glycemic index, glycemic load, and risk of type 2 diabetes. Am J Clin Nutr 2002;76:274S–80S.

Yaffe K, Blackwell T, Kanaya AM, Davidowitz N, Barrett-Connor E, Krueger K. Diabetes, impaired fasting glucose, and development of cognitive impairment in older women. Neurology 2004;63:658–63.

Yaffe K, Kanaya A, Lindquist K, et al. The metabolic syndrome, inflammation, and risk of cognitive decline. JAMA 2004;292:2237–42.

Yusuf N, Irby C, Katiyar SK, Elmets CA. Photoprotective effects of green tea polyphenols. Photodermat Photo 2007;23:48–56.
Zoeller RFJR. Physical activity and obesity: their interaction and implications for disease
 risk and the role of physical activity in healthy weight management. American Journal
 of Lifestyle Medicine 2007;1:437–46.

## Chapter 4

American Medical Association. AMA calls for measures to reduce sodium intake in U.S.
 diet. In: www.ama-assn.org/ama/pub/category/16461.html; 2006.
Authors/Task Force M, Mancia G, De Backer G, et al. 2007 Guidelines for the manage-
 ment of arterial hypertension: The Task Force for the Management of Arterial
 Hypertension of the European Society of Hypertension (ESH) and of the European
 Society of Cardiology (ESC). Eur Heart J 2007;28:1462–536.
Bacopa monniera. Monograph. Altern Med Rev 2004;9:79–85.
Block G, Jensen C, Norkus E, et al. Usage patterns, health, and nutritional status of
 long-term multiple dietary supplement users: a cross-sectional study. Nutr J 2007;6:30.
Boushey CJ, Beresford SA, Omenn GS, Motulsky AG. A quantitative assessment of
 plasma homocysteine as a risk factor for vascular disease. Probable benefits of
 increasing folic acid intakes. [See comment.] JAMA 1995;274:1049–57.
Chavarro JE, Rich-Edwards JW, Rosner BA, Willett WC. Use of multivitamins, intake
 of B vitamins, and risk of ovulatory infertility. Fertil Steril 2008;89:668–76.
Clarke R. Homocysteine-lowering vitamin B supplements do not improve cognitive per-
 formance in healthy older adults after two years. Evid Based Ment Health 2007;10:27.
Clarke R, Birks J, Nexo E, et al. Low vitamin B-12 status and risk of cognitive decline in
 older adults. Am J Clin Nutr 2007;86:1384–91.
Corrada MM, Kawas CH, Hallfrisch J, Muller D, Brookmeyer R. Reduced risk of
 Alzheimer's disease with high folate intake: the Baltimore Longitudinal Study of
 Aging. Alzheimer's and Dementia. Journal of the Alzheimer's Association 2005;1:11–8.
DeKosky ST, Williamson JD, Fitzpatrick AL, et al. Ginkgo biloba for prevention of
 dementia: a randomized controlled trial. JAMA 2008;300:2253–62.
de Lau LML, Refsum H, Smith AD, Johnston C, Breteler MMB. Plasma folate
 concentration and cognitive performance: Rotterdam Scan Study. Am J Clin Nutr
 2007;86:728–34.
Dietary Reference Intakes for Energy, Carbohydrate, Fiber, Fat, Fatty Acids, Cholesterol,
 Protein, and Amino Acids (2002). National Academy of Sciences Copyright 2002 by
 the National Academy of Sciences. All rights reserved, 2002. www.nap.edu.
Dietary Supplement Fact Sheet: Folate. National Institutes of Health, 2004. www.ods.
 od.nih.gov/factsheets/folate.asp.
Dietary Supplement Fact Sheet: Vitamin B12. National Institutes of Health. Office of
 Dietary Supplements, 2002. www.ods.od.nih.gov/factsheets/vitaminb12.asp.
Durga J, Verhoef P, Anteunis LJC, Schouten E, Kok FJ. Effects of folic acid supplemen-
 tation on hearing in older adults: a randomized, controlled trial. [See comment.]

[Summary for patients in Ann Intern Med 2007 Jan 2;146(1):I20; PMID: 17200213.] Ann Intern Med 2007;146:1–9.

Engelhart MJ, Geerlings MI, Ruitenberg A, et al. Dietary intake of antioxidants and risk of Alzheimer disease. [See comment.] JAMA 2002;287:3223–9.

Facts about Dietary Supplements. Vitamin B6. National Institutes of Health. Office of Dietary Supplements, 2002. wwwods.od.nih.gov/factsheets/cc/vitb6.html.

Fanjiang G, Kleinman RE. Nutrition and performance in children. [Miscellaneous.] Curr Opin Clin Nutr May 2007;10:342–7.

Figueiredo JC, Levine AJ, Grau MV, et al. Vitamins B2, B6, and B12 and risk of new colorectal adenomas in a randomized trial of aspirin use and folic acid supplementation. Cancer Epidem Biomar 2008;17:2136–45.

Giovannucci E. Can vitamin D reduce total mortality? Arch Intern Med 2007;167:1709–10.

Godfrey JR. Toward optimal health: Meir Stampfer, M.D., Dr.P.H., discusses multivitamin and mineral supplementation for women. J Women's Health 2007;16:959–62.

Gonzalez S, Huerta JM, Fernandez S, Patterson AM, Lasheras C. Homocysteine increases the risk of mortality in elderly individuals. Brit J Nutrition 2007;97:1138–43.

Gray SL, Anderson ML, Crane PK, et al. Antioxidant vitamin supplement use and risk of dementia or Alzheimer's disease in older adults. J Am Geriat Soc 2008;56:291–5.

Haan MN, Miller JW, Aiello AE, et al. Homocysteine, B vitamins, and the incidence of dementia and cognitive impairment: results from the Sacramento Area Latino Study on Aging. Am J Clin Nutr 2007;85:511–7.

Harding A-H, Wareham NJ, Bingham SA, et al. Plasma vitamin C level, fruit and vegetable consumption, and the risk of new-onset type 2 diabetes mellitus: the European Prospective Investigation of Cancer-Norfolk Prospective Study. Arch Intern Med 2008;168:1493–9.

Havas S, Roccella EJ, Lenfant C. Reducing the public health burden from elevated blood pressure levels in the United States by lowering intake of dietary sodium. Am J Public Health 2004;94:19–22.

Hickey S, Noriega L, Roberts H. Re: multivitamin use and risk of prostate cancer in the National Institutes of Health AARP Diet and Health Study. J Natl Cancer I 2007;99:1491–2.

Hin H, Clarke R, Sherliker P, et al. Clinical relevance of low serum vitamin B12 concentrations in older people: the Banbury B12 study. Age Ageing 2006;35:416–22.

Holick MF. High prevalence of vitamin D inadequacy and implications for health. [See comment.] Mayo Clin Proc 2006;81:353–73.

Holick MF. Vitamin D deficiency. New Engl J Med 2007;357:266–81.

Hollis BW, Wagner CL. Vitamin D deficiency during pregnancy: an ongoing epidemic. Am J Clin Nutr 2006;84:273.

Hoogendijk WJG, Lips P, Dik MG, Deeg DJH, Beekman ATF, Penninx BWJH. Depression is associated with decreased 25-hydroxyvitamin D and increased parathyroid hormone levels in older adults. Arch Gen Psychiat 2008;65:508–12.

Hudson S, Tabet N. Acetyl-L-carnitine for dementia. Cochrane Db Syst Rev 2003:CD003158.

Hypponen E, Power C. Hypovitaminosis D in British adults at age 45 y: nationwide cohort study of dietary and lifestyle predictors. Am J Clin Nutr 2007;85:860–8.

Institute of Medicine. Dietary reference intakes: water, potassium, sodium, chloride, and sulfate. Washington, DC: National Academies Press; 2004.

Institute of Medicine of the National Academies. Dietary Reference Intakes for Water, Potassium, Sodium, Chloride, and Sulfate. Washington DC: National Academies Press; 2005.

Ishihara J, Iso H, Inoue M, et al. Intake of folate, vitamin B6 and vitamin B12 and the risk of CHD: the Japan Public Health Center-Based Prospective Study Cohort I. J Am Coll Nutr 2008;27:127–36.

Ishitani K, Lin J, Manson JE, Buring JE, Zhang SM. A prospective study of multivitamin supplement use and risk of breast cancer. Am J Epidem 2008;167:1197–206.

Jacobsen MF, Hurley JG, Center for Science in the Public Interest. Restaurant Confidential. New York: Workman Publishing; 2002.

Kim J, Park MH, Kim E, Han C, Jo SA, Jo I. Plasma homocysteine is associated with the risk of mild cognitive impairment in an elderly Korean population. J Nutr 2007;137:2093–7.

Kim JM, Stewart R, Kim SW, et al. Changes in folate, vitamin B12 and homocysteine associated with incident dementia. J Neurol Neurosur Ps 2008;79:864–8.

Kretsch MJ, Fong AK, Green MW, Johnson HL. Cognitive function, iron status, and hemoglobin concentration in obese dieting women. Eur J Clin Nutr 1998;52:512–8.

Kretsch MJ, Green MW, Fong AK, Elliman NA, Johnson HL. Cognitive effects of a long-term weight reducing diet. Int J Obes Relat Metab Disord, Journal of the International Association for the Study of Obesity 1997;21:14–21.

Lappe JM, Travers-Gustafson D, Davies KM, Recker RR, Heaney RP. Vitamin D and calcium supplementation reduces cancer risk: results of a randomized trial. Am J Clin Nutr 2007;85:1586–91.

Lawson KA, Wright ME, Subar A, et al. Multivitamin use and risk of prostate cancer in the National Institutes of Health–AARP Diet and Health Study. J Natl Cancer I 2007;99:754–64.

Liu S, Song Y, Ford ES, Manson JE, Buring JE, Ridker PM. Dietary calcium, vitamin D, and the prevalence of metabolic syndrome in middle-aged and older U.S. women. Diabetes Care 2005;28:2926–32.

Louwman MW, van Dusseldorp M, van de Vijver FJ, et al. Signs of impaired cognitive function in adolescents with marginal cobalamin status. A J Clin Nutr 2000;72:762–9.

Luchsinger JA, Tang M-X, Miller J, Green R, Mayeux R. Relation of higher folate intake to lower risk of Alzheimer disease in the elderly. Arch Neurol 2007;64:86–92.

Machlin LJ, ed. Handbook of Vitamins. 2nd ed. New York: Marcel Dekker; 1991.

Magnesium. National Institutes of Health, 2005. www.dietary-supplements.info.nih.gov/factsheets/magnesium.asp.

Mahan KL, Arlin M. Krause's Food, Nutrition & Diet Therapy. 8th ed. Philadelphia: W. B. Saunders Co.; 1992.

Martins D, Wolf M, Pan D, et al. Prevalence of cardiovascular risk factors and the serum levels of 25-hydroxyvitamin D in the United States: data from the Third National Health and Nutrition Examination Survey. Arch Intern Med 2007;167:1159–65.

Mattes RD, Donnelly D. Relative contributions of dietary sodium sources. J Am Coll Nutr 1991;10:383–93.

Melamed ML, Michos ED, Post W, Astor B. 25-Hydroxyvitamin D levels and the risk of
    mortality in the general population. Arch Intern Med 2008;168:1629–37.

Morris MC, Evans DA, Bienias JL, et al. Dietary niacin and the risk of incident
    Alzheimer's disease and of cognitive decline. J Neurol Neurosur Ps 2004;75:1093–9.

Morris MS, Jacques PF, Rosenberg IH, Selhub J. Hyperhomocysteinemia associated with
    poor recall in the third National Health and Nutrition Examination Survey. Am J
    Clin Nutr 2001;73:927–33.

Munger K, Zhang S, O'Reilly E, et al. Vitamin D intake and incidence of multiple
    sclerosis. Neurology 2004;62:60–5.

National Center for Complementary and Alternative medicine. Ginkgo NCCAM
    Publication No. D290. In: Herbs at a Glance, National Institutes of Health,
    National Center for Complementary and Alternative Medicine, Department of
    Health & Human Services; 2008.

O'Sullivan M, Nic Suibhne T, Cox G, Healy M, O'Morain C. High prevalence of
    vitamin D insufficiency in healthy Irish adults. Irish J Med Sci 2008;177:131–4.

Pang Z, Pan F, He S. Ginkgo biloba L.: history, current status, and future prospects.
    [Erratum appears in J Altern Complement Med 1997 Summer;3(2):205.] J Altern
    Complement Med 1996;2:359–63.

Pittas AG, Harris SS, Stark PC, Dawson-Hughes B. The effects of calcium and vitamin
    D supplementation on blood glucose and markers of inflammation in nondiabetic
    adults. Diabetes Care 2007;30:980–6.

Pittas AG, Lau J, Hu FB, Dawson-Hughes B. The role of vitamin D and calcium
    in type 2 diabetes. A systematic review and meta-analysis. J Clin Endocr Metab
    2007;92:2017–29.

Quadri P, Fragiacomo C, Pezzati R, et al. Homocysteine, folate, and vitamin B-12 in
    mild cognitive impairment, Alzheimer disease, and vascular dementia. Am J Clin
    Nutr 2004;80:114–22.

Ramos MI, Allen LH, Mungas DM, et al. Low folate status is associated with impaired
    cognitive function and dementia in the Sacramento Area Latino Study on Aging. Am
    J Clin Nutr 2005;82:1346–52.

Ravaglia G, Forti P, Maioli F, et al. Homocysteine and folate as risk factors for dementia
    and Alzheimer disease. Am J Clin Nutr 2005;82:636–43.

A Report of the Standing Committee on the Scientific Evaluation of Dietary Reference
    Intakes and Its Panel on Folate OBV, and Choline and Subcommittee on Upper
    Reference Levels of Nutrients, Food and Nutrition Board, Institute of Medicine.
    Dietary Reference Intakes for Thiamin, Riboflavin, Niacin, Vitamin B6, Folate,
    Vitamin B12, Pantothenic Acid, Biotin, and Choline. Washington DC: National
    Academy Press; 1998.

Russo A, Borrelli F. Bacopa monniera, a reputed nootropic plant: an overview.
    Phytomedicine 2005;12:305–17.

Scouting for Sodium. And Other Nutrients Important to Blood Pressure. 1994. www.fda.
    gov/fdac/foodlabel/sodium.html.

Seshadri S, Beiser A, Selhub J, et al. Plasma homocysteine as a risk factor for dementia
    and Alzheimer's disease.[See Comment]. New Eng. J. Med. 2002;346:476–83.

Shurin S Dr. Vitamin B12—State of the Science. Washington DC: House Committee on Oversight and Government Reform, U.S. Department of Health & Human Services; 2008.

Soinio M, Marniemi J, Laakso M, Lehto S, Ronnemaa T. Elevated plasma homocysteine level is an independent predictor of coronary heart disease events in patients with type 2 diabetes mellitus. Ann Intern Med 2004;140:94–100.

Son Y-J. Hostility and serum homocysteine as cardiovascular risk factors in Korean patients with coronary artery disease. J Clin Nurs 2007;16:672–8.

Spinneker A, Sola R, Lemmen V, Castillo MJ, Pietrzik K, Gonzalez-Gross M. Vitamin B6 status, deficiency and its consequences—an overview. Nutricion Hospitalaria 2007;22:7–24.

Stehouwer CDA, Weijenberg MP, van den Berg M, Jakobs C, Feskens EJM, Kromhout D. Serum homocysteine and risk of coronary heart disease and cerebrovascular disease in elderly men: a 10-year follow-up. Arterioscl Throm Vas 1998;18:1895–901.

Tanne D, Haim M, Goldbourt U, et al. Prospective study of serum homocysteine and risk of ischemic stroke among patients with preexisting coronary heart disease. Stroke 2003;34:632–6.

Tröhler U. James Lind and Scurvy. In: The James Lind Library. www.jameslindlibrary .org; 2003.

USDA Center for Nutrition Policy and Promotion. Insight 3: Dietary Guidance on Sodium Should We Take It with a Grain of Salt? Center for Nutrition Policy and Promotion; 1997 May.

USDA National Nutrient Database for Standard Reference. Release 20. United States Department of Agriculture. Agricultural Research Service, 2007. www.ars.usda.gov/ ba/bhnrc/ndl.

van der Meer IM, Karamali NS, Boeke AJP, et al. High prevalence of vitamin D deficiency in pregnant non-Western women in The Hague, Netherlands. Am J Clin Nutr 2006;84:350–3.

Vieth R, Bischoff-Ferrari H, Boucher BJ, et al. The urgent need to recommend an intake of vitamin D that is effective. Am J Clin Nutr 2007;85:649–50.

Waife SO. Lind, lemons and limeys. Am J Clin Nutr 1953;1:471–3.

Wilkins CH, Sheline YI, Roe CM, Birge SJ, Morris JC. Vitamin D deficiency is associated with low mood and worse cognitive performance in older adults. Am J Geriat Psychiat 2006;14:1032–40. www.cspinet.org/new/pdf/cspirestaurantsaltreport.pdf.

www.pagebypagebooks.com/Hugh_Lofting/The_Story_of_Doctor_Dolittle/ The_Rarest_Animal_Of_All_p1.html.

Zandi PP, Anthony JC, Khachaturian AS, et al. Reduced risk of Alzheimer disease in users of antioxidant vitamin supplements: the Cache County Study. Arch Neurol 2004;61:82–8.

Zhang SM, Moore SC, Lin J, et al. Folate, vitamin B6, multivitamin supplements, and colorectal cancer risk in women. Am J Epidem 2006;163:108–15.

## Chapter 5

Abbott RD, White LR, Ross GW, Masaki KH, Curb JD, Petrovitch H. Walking and dementia in physically capable elderly men. JAMA 2004;292:1447–53.

Beydoun MA, Beydoun HA, Wang Y. Obesity and central obesity as risk factors for incident dementia and its subtypes: a systematic review and meta-analysis. [Erratum appears in Obes Rev 2008 May;9(3):267]. Obes Rev 2008;9:204–18.

Bigaard J, Frederiksen K, Tjonneland A, et al. Waist circumference and body composition in relation to all-cause mortality in middle-aged men and women. Int J Obes Relat Metab Disord 2005;29:778–84.

Carlson SA, Fulton JE, Lee SM, et al. Physical education and academic achievement in elementary school: data from the Early Childhood Longitudinal Study. Am J Public Health 2008;98:721–7.

Cassilhas RC, Viana VAR, Grassmann V, et al. The impact of resistance exercise on the cognitive function of the elderly. Medicine & Science in Sports & Exercise 2007;39:1401–7.

Centers for Disease Control. Obesity Still a Major Problem. In: National Center for Health Statistics: U.S. Department of Health and Human Services; 2007.

Cherkas LF, Hunkin JL, Kato BS, et al. The association between physical activity in leisure time and leukocyte telomere length. Arch Intern Med 2008;168:154–8.

Cleland VJ, Schmidt MD, Dwyer T, Venn AJ. Television viewing and abdominal obesity in young adults: is the association mediated by food and beverage consumption during viewing time or reduced leisure-time physical activity? Am J Clin Nutr 2008;87:1148–55.

Colcombe SJ, Erickson KI, Raz N, et al. Aerobic fitness reduces brain tissue loss in aging humans. J Gerontol A Biol Sci Med Sci 2003;58:M176–80.

Colcombe SJ, Kramer AF, Erickson KI, et al. Cardiovascular fitness, cortical plasticity, and aging. Proceedings of the National Academy of Sciences of the United States of America 2004;101:3316–21.

Couillard C, Ruel G, Archer WR, et al. Circulating levels of oxidative stress markers and endothelial adhesion molecules in men with abdominal obesity. J Clin Endocr Metab 2005;90:6454–9.

Dorn JM, Hovey K, Muti P, et al. Alcohol drinking patterns differentially affect central adiposity as measured by abdominal height in women and men. J Nutr 2003;133:2655–62.

Epel ESP, McEwen BP, Seeman TP, et al. Stress and body shape: stress-induced cortisol secretion is consistently greater among women with central fat. Psychosomatic Medicine 2000;62:623–32.

Ertel KA, Glymour MM, Berkman LF. Effects of social integration on preserving memory function in a nationally representative US elderly population. Am J Public Health 2008;98:1215–20.

Expert Panel on Detection E, Treatment of High Blood Cholesterol in A. Executive Summary of the Third Report of the National Cholesterol Education Program

(NCEP) Expert Panel on Detection, Evaluation, and Treatment of High Blood Cholesterol in Adults (Adult Treatment Panel III). JAMA 2001;285:2486–97.

Ferris LT, Williams JS, Shen C-L. The effect of acute exercise on serum brain-derived neurotrophic factor levels and cognitive function. Medicine & Science in Sports & Exercise 2007;39:728–34.

Fontana L, Eagon JC, Trujillo ME, Scherer PE, Klein S. Visceral fat adipokine secretion is associated with systemic inflammation in obese humans. Diabetes 2007;56:1010–3.

Fratiglioni L, Paillard-Borg S, Winblad B. An active and socially integrated lifestyle in late life might protect against dementia. Lancet Neurology 2004;3:343–53.

Janz KF, Levy SM, Burns TL, Torner JC, Willing MC, Warren JJ. Fatness, physical activity, and television viewing in children during the adiposity rebound period: The Iowa Bone Development Study. Preventive Medicine 2002;35:563–71.

Javaheri S, Storfer-Isser A, Rosen CL, Redline S. Sleep quality and elevated blood pressure in adolescents. Circulation 2008;118:1034–40.

Kanai H, Matsuzawa Y, Kotani K, et al. Close correlation of intra-abdominal fat accumulation to hypertension in obese women. Hypertension 1990;16:484–90.

Larson EB, Wang L, Bowen JD, et al. Exercise is associated with reduced risk for incident dementia among persons 65 years of age and older. Ann Intern Med 2006;144:73–81.

Lautenschlager NT, Cox KL, Flicker L, et al. Effect of physical activity on cognitive function in older adults at risk for Alzheimer disease: a randomized trial. JAMA 2008;300:1027–37.

Lee C-D, Jacobs DR, Jr., Schreiner PJ, Iribarren C, Hankinson A. Abdominal obesity and coronary artery calcification in young adults: the Coronary Artery Risk Development in Young Adults (CARDIA) Study. Am J Clin Nutr 2007;86:48–54.

Lemieux I, Pascot A, Prud'homme D, et al. Elevated C-reactive protein: another component of the atherothrombotic profile of abdominal obesity. [See comment.] Arterioscl Throm Vas 2001;21:961–7.

Lopez-Garcia E, Faubel R, Leon-Munoz L, Zuluaga MC, Banegas JR, Rodriguez-Artalejo F. Sleep duration, general and abdominal obesity, and weight change among the older adult population of Spain. Am J Clin Nutr 2008;87:310–6.

Luft AR, Macko RF, Forrester LW, et al. Treadmill exercise activates subcortical neural networks and improves walking after stroke. A Randomized Controlled Trial. Stroke 2008;39:3341–50.

Lumeng JC, Rahnama S, Appugliese D, Kaciroti N, Bradley RH. Television exposure and overweight risk in preschoolers. Arch Pediatr Adolesc Med 2006;160:417–22.

Lytle ME, Vander Bilt J, Pandav RS, Dodge HH, Ganguli M. Exercise level and cognitive decline: the MoVIES project. [See comment.] Alzheimer Disease & Associated Disorders 2004;18:57–64.

Matsuzawa Y. Therapy Insight: adipocytokines in metabolic syndrome and related cardiovascular disease. Nature Clinical Practice Cardiovascular Medicine 2006;3:35–42.

McAuley E, Kramer AF, Colcombe SJ. Cardiovascular fitness and neurocognitive function in older adults: a brief review. Brain, Behavior, and Immunity 2004;18:214.

Melov S, Tarnopolsky MA, Beckman K, Felkey K, Hubbard A. Resistance exercise reverses aging in human skeletal muscle. PLoS One 2007;2:e465.

Merchant AT, Anand SS, Vuksan V, et al. Protein intake is inversely associated with abdominal obesity in a multi-ethnic population. J Nutr 2005;135:1196–201.

Metcalf BS, Voss LD, Hosking J, Jeffery AN, Wilkin TJ. Physical activity at the government-recommended level and obesity-related health outcomes: a longitudinal study (Early Bird 37). Arch Dis Child 2008;93:772–7.

Mukherjee Debabrata. News from the American Stroke Association's International Stroke Conference 2008, New Orleans, La., February 20–22, 2008. In: Cardiology Review Newsbeat. Plainsboro; 2008.

National Sleep Foundation. 2008 Sleep in America Poll. Summary of Findings; 2008 March. Report No.: Job #07-139.

Newson RS, Kemps EB. Cardiorespiratory fitness as a predictor of successful cognitive ageing. J Clin Exp Neuropsych 2006;28:949–67.

Pou KM, Massaro JM, Hoffmann U, et al. Visceral and subcutaneous adipose tissue volumes are cross-sectionally related to markers of inflammation and oxidative stress: the Framingham Heart Study. Circulation 2007;116:1234–41.

The Problem of Overweight in Children and Adolescents. U.S. Department of Health & Human Services, 2007. www.surgeongeneral.gov/topics/obesity/calltoaction/fact_adolescents.htm.

Slentz CA, Aiken LB, Houmard JA, et al. Inactivity, exercise, and visceral fat. STRRIDE: a randomized, controlled study of exercise intensity and amount. J of Applied Physiology 2005;99:1613–8.

Strong WB, Malina RM, Blimkie CJR, et al. Evidence based physical activity for school-age youth. [See comment.] J Pediat 2005;146:732–7.

U.S. Department of Health and Human Services, National Institutes of Health, National Heart Lung and Blood Institute. Your Guide to A Healthy Sleep. Washington, DC; 2005 November. Report No.: NIH Publication No. 06-5271.

von Hafe P, Pina F, Perez A, Tavares M, Barros H. Visceral fat accumulation as a risk factor for prostate cancer. Obes Res 2004;12:1930–5.

Wang JYJ, Zhou DHD, Li J, et al. Leisure activity and risk of cognitive impairment: the Chongqing aging study. [See comment.] Neurology 2006;66:911–3.

Wang Y, Rimm EB, Stampfer MJ, Willett WC, Hu FB. Comparison of abdominal adiposity and overall obesity in predicting risk of type 2 diabetes among men. Am J Clin Nutr 2005;81:555–63.

Weuve J, Kang JH, Manson JE, Breteler MMB, Ware JH, Grodstein F. Physical activity, including walking, and cognitive function in older women. JAMA 2004;292:1454–61.

Whitbourne SB, Neupert SD, Lachman ME. Daily Physical Activity: Relation to everyday memory in adulthood. J Appl Gerontol 2008;27:331–49.

Whitmer RA, Gustafson DR, Barrett-Connor E, Haan MN, Gunderson EP, Yaffe K. Central obesity and increased risk of dementia more than three decades later. Neurology 2008;71:1057–64.

Wildman RP, Muntner P, Reynolds K, et al. The obese without cardiometabolic risk factor clustering and the normal weight with cardiometabolic risk factor clustering: prevalence and correlates of 2 phenotypes among the US population (NHANES 1999–2004). Arch Intern Med 2008;168:1617–24.

Wilson RS, Scherr PA, Schneider JA, Tang Y, Bennett DA. Relation of cognitive activity to risk of developing Alzheimer disease. Neurology 2007;69:1911–20.

Winter B, Breitenstein C, Mooren FC, et al. High impact running improves learning. Neurobiology of Learning and Memory 2007;87:597–609.

Winter Y, Rohrmann S, Linseisen J, et al. Contribution of obesity and abdominal fat
   mass to risk of stroke and transient ischemic sttacks. Stroke 2008;39:3145–51.
Zhang C, Rexrode KM, van Dam RM, Li TY, Hu FB. Abdominal obesity and the risk
   of all-cause, cardiovascular, and cancer mortality: sixteen years of follow-up in US
   women. Circulation 2008;117:1658–67.

# Chapter 6

Fredholm Bertil B, Battig K, Holmen J, Nehlig A, Zvartau EE. Actions of caffeine in
   the brain with special reference to factors that contribute to its widespread use.
   Pharmacol Rev 1999;51:83 133.
Gunzerath L, Faden V, Zakhari S, Warren K. National Institute on Alcohol Abuse
   and Alcoholism report on moderate drinking. Alcoholism: Clinical & Experimental
   Research 2004;28:829–47.
Johnson-Kozlow M, Kritz-Silverstein D, Barrett-Connor E, Morton D. Coffee consump-
   tion and cognitive function among older adults. Am J Epidem 2002;156:842–50.
Malinauskas B, Aeby V, Overton R, Carpenter-Aeby T, Barber-Heidal K. A survey of
   energy drink consumption patterns among college students. Nutr J 2007;6:35.
McLellan TM, Kamimori GH, Voss DM, Tate C, Smith SJR. Caffeine effects on
   physical and cognitive performance during sustained operations. Aviation, Space, and
   Environmental Medicine 2007;78:871–7.
Mehlig K, Skoog I, Guo X, et al. Alcoholic beverages and incidence of dementia: 34-year
   follow-up of the prospective population study of women in Goteborg. Am J Epidem
   2008;167:684–91.
Mukamal KJ, Kuller LH, Fitzpatrick AL, Longstreth WT, Jr., Mittleman MA, Siscovick
   DS. Prospective study of alcohol consumption and risk of dementia in older adults.
   JAMA 2003;289:1405–13.
O'Keefe JH, Bybee KA, Lavie CJ. Alcohol and cardiovascular health: The razor-sharp
   double-edged sword. J Am Coll Cardiol 2007;50:1009–14.
Peters R, Peters J, Warner J, Beckett N, Bulpitt C. Alcohol, dementia and cognitive
   decline in the elderly: a systematic review. Age Ageing 2008;37:505–12.
Ritchie K, Carriere I, de Mendonca A, et al. The neuroprotective effects of caffeine: a
   prospective population study (the Three City Study). Neurology 2007;69:536–45.
Solfrizzi V, D'Introno A, Colacicco AM, et al. Alcohol consumption, mild cognitive
   impairment, and progression to dementia. Neurology 2007;68:1790–9.
Stampfer MJ, Kang JH, Chen J, Cherry R, Grodstein F. Effects of moderate alcohol
   consumption on cognitive function in women. [See Comment]. New Engl J Med
   2005;352:245–53.

## Chapter 8

American Pain Foundation. Pain Facts & Figures. In: wwwpainfoundationorg/
    pageasp?file=Newsroom/PainFactshtm; 2007.
Bazzano LA, Song Y, Bubes V, Good CK, Manson JE, Liu S. Dietary intake of
    whole and refined grain breakfast cereals and weight gain in men. Obesity Res
    2005;13:1952–60.
The Better Sleep Council. When Should I Replace My Mattress? In: www.bettersleep.
    org/OnBetterSleep/when_to_replace.asp, 2007.
Bowen D, Fesinmeyer M, Yasui Y, et al. Randomized trial of exercise in sedentary middle
    aged women: effects on quality of life. Int J Behav Nutr Phy 2006;3:34.
Hamer M, Stamatakis E, Steptoe A. Dose response relationship between physical activity
    and mental health: The Scottish Health Survey. Brit J Sports Med 2008 doi:10.1136/
    bjsm.2008.046243 published online 10 Apr 2008.
Hansen CJ, Stevens LC, Coast JR. Exercise duration and mood state: how much is
    enough to feel better? Health Psychology 2001;20:267–75.
Ingwersen J, Defeyter MA, Kennedy DO, Wesnes KA, Scholey AB. Influence of breakfast
    composition next term on children's attention and memory. Appetite 2006;47:267.
Ingwersen J, Defeyter MA, Kennedy DO, Wesnes KA, Scholey AB. A low glycaemic
    index breakfast cereal preferentially prevents children's cognitive performance from
    declining throughout the morning. Appetite 2007;49:240–4.
Jacobson BH, Wallace TJ, Smith DB, Kolb T. Grouped comparisons of sleep quality for
    new and personal bedding systems. Applied Ergonomics 2008;39:247–54.
Kleinman RE, Hall S, Green H, et al. Diet, breakfast, and academic performance in
    children. Ann Nutr Metab 2002;46 Suppl 1:24–30.
Kovacs FM, Abraira V, PeÒa A, et al. Effect of firmness of mattress on chronic
    non-specific low-back pain: randomised, double-blind, controlled, multicentre trial.
    Lancet 2003;362:1599–604.
Mahoney CR, Taylor HA, Kanarek RB, Samuel P. Effect of breakfast composition on
    cognitive processes in elementary school children. Physiol Behav 2005;85:635–45.
Teychenne M, Ball K, Salmon J. Associations between physical activity and depressive
    symptoms in women. Int J Behavi Nutr Phy 2008;5:27.
Ybarra O, Burnstein E, Winkielman P, et al. Mental exercising through simple social-
    izing: social interaction promotes general cognitive functioning. Pers Soc Psychol
    Bull 2008;34:248–59.

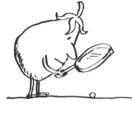

# Index